129,
130

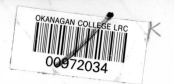
| DATE DUE | | |
|---|---|---|
| OCT 2 9 1981 | OCT 1 9 1993 | Reg - 762913714 |
| FEB 0 3 1982 | APR 9 1994 | |
| MAR 0 5 1982 | DEC - 2 1995 | |
| MAR 1 1985 | NOV 1 2 1996 | |
| JUN 2 2 1988 | APR 1 0 1997 | |
| | JAN 2 1 1999 | |
| FEB 5 1990 | March 12/99 | |
| FEB 1 9 1990 | SEP 3 0 1998 | |
| MAR 1 4 1990 | NOV 1 5 2000 | |
| MAR 2 8 1990 | OCT 1 1 2001 | |
| APR 1 1 1990 | NOV 2 0 2001 | |
| FEB 1 6 1990 | FEB - 7 2002 | |
| | NOV 1 2 | |

**MURIEL FFOULKES L.R.C.**
**OKANAGAN COLLEGE**
**British Columbia**
**V1Y 4X8**

# THE SCIENTIFIC REVOLUTION IN
# VICTORIAN MEDICINE

# The Scientific Revolution in Victorian Medicine

A. J. YOUNGSON

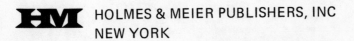 HOLMES & MEIER PUBLISHERS, INC
NEW YORK

PRINTED IN GREAT BRITAIN
First published in the United States of America 1979 by
HOLMES & MEIER PUBLISHERS, INC.
30 Irving Place, New York, N.Y. 10003

Copyright © 1979 A. J. Youngson

**Library of Congress Cataloging in Publication Data**

Youngson, A J
    The scientific revolution in Victorian medicine.

    Bibliography: p.
    Includes index.
    1. Medicine – Great Britain – History – 19th century.
2. Surgery – Great Britain – History – 19th century.
3. Medical innovations – Great Britain – History 19th
century.  I.  Title.  [DNLM:  1. History of medicine,
19th Century – England.  WZ70 FE5 Y8s]
R487. Y68      610'. 941      78–31705
ISBN 0–8419–0479–0

# CONTENTS

*In memoriam* Alexander Brown, MB  ChB

# PREFACE

This book is a study of the resistance to new ideas. Such resistance is encountered not only in medicine, but probably in every field of human thought and endeavour. Because new ideas are the fuel of progress, we are apt to assume that those who resist new ideas are dull or obscurantist, or that they have a vested interest in the *status quo*; and such may often be the case. We are also apt to assume that those who resisted new ideas which time has proved to be valuable must have been seriously mistaken. But this need not be so. For us, accustomed to innumerable ideas and devices which once were new, there is no shock in them of novelty; their success is plain to see; such deficiencies as they originally contained have long been made good. But that is not how it was at the time, and therefore the opposition to new ideas may not be unreasonable, even to ideas which triumph in the end. To dismiss such opposition as stupid or absurd is to fail to understand how ideas conflict and develop, and how progress really takes place.

My work would have been impossible without the help of several institutions and of many more persons. The Australian National University, which enabled me to visit the United Kingdom in 1978 in order to gather material not available in Australia; the Royal College of Physicians of Edinburgh, and the Royal College of Surgeons of Edinburgh, who most kindly allowed me access to their libraries and whose libraries gave me courteous, valuable and expert assistance; and the University of Edinburgh, the library of which was also most generously made available to me. Of those who gave encouragement and advice, I am especially indebted to Professor A.S. Duncan, Professor W. Hayes, and Dr G.I.M. Ross, each of whom read a part of the typescript. They may not wish to be associated with the final result, and are certainly in no way responsible for the errors and omissions which the following pages may contain.

Finally, I wish to express my thanks, yet again, to my wife, whose skill in indexing and proof-reading very far exceeds my own.

Canberra December 1978

# 1 MEDICINE AND SURGERY IN EARLY VICTORIAN BRITAIN

Knowledge is power; more specifically, scientific knowledge is power. This idea, put forward with magniloquent authority by Francis Bacon early in the seventeenth century and reiterated and elaborated by many subsequent writers, is the foundation of the modern world.

The connection — and we need not doubt that a connection exists — between science and power and technology, and between technology and higher living standards, and between higher living standards and progress that really is progress, is long and intricate and difficult to determine. But years ago the path that connects science with progress seemed, to those who had scarcely begun to travel along it, a broad highway, and the conviction spread that science not only leads to progress, but virtually guarantees it. Largely as a result of this opinion, those who then studied man's history and who speculated about his future were, on the whole, more hopeful than anyone had been before, and than anyone has been since. It was felt no longer necessary to imagine paradise as existing only in the hereafter, or in the form of an antique golden age or a state of nature long past. The new faith was that paradise lay in the future. In the future, wrote Joseph Priestley in 1768.

> all knowledge will be subdivided and extended; and knowledge, as Lord Bacon observes, being power, the human powers will, in fact, be increased; nature, including both its materials, and its laws, will be more at our command; men will make their situation in this world abundantly more easy and comfortable; they will probably prolong their existence in it, and will grow daily more happy, each in himself, and more able (and, I believe, more disposed) to communicate happiness to others.[1]

The contemplation of this prospect 'always makes me happy' he added.

Priestley died shortly after 1800. In the next three or four decades changes took place which seemed to suggest that his vision might be realised. In science and technology remarkable progress had been and continued to be made, and the flow of discovery became stronger and stronger as the years passed. Priestley himself was the discoverer of oxygen, and of the absorption of carbon dioxide by chlorophyll in sunlight; and as a young man he had carried out a series of brilliant if slipshod experiments in electricity and had written a *History of Electricity* for which he was made a Fellow of the Royal Society. A close contemporary, Lavoisier, founded the modern theory of the chemical elements and began the modern science of quantitative organic analysis. His work destroyed the prevalent idea, which medieval alchemists would have recognised, that substances in general contain three constituents, one of them a mysterious 'spirit' (possibly having negative weight) which could be liberated by heating. Another close contemporary, James Watt, discovered the composition of water, and as a result of careful work on the relation between the temperature and pressure of steam, made improvements to the steam engine which changed it from a barely useful device into the principal agent in the creation of modern industry and transport. Sir Humphry Davy discovered potassium, sodium and nitrous oxide, demonstrated the elementary nature of chlorine and, a few years after Priestley's death published *Elements of Agricultural Chemistry*, a book which completely superseded all previous publications on the subject and continued as a standard work for fifty years. This list might be greatly extended. But what is important is not only the number of discoveries made, but equally the path-breaking and even the epoch-making character of many of them.

For it was on the basis of these and other scientific and technical advances that a new generation of engineers, businessmen, farmers and bankers brought about changes of unparalleled speed and extent which affected the lives of men and women in all walks of life. The new order of things first took shape in Britain. Not in a few years, but certainly in a few decades, Britain altered from being a largely traditional, agricultural, aristocratic society into one in which science, innovation and industry increasingly set the pace. Nothing like this had ever happened before, and to begin with nothing like it was happening anywhere else. One of the most distinguished economists and historians of his day was Simonde de Sismondi. He visited England in the 1820s and in the opening lines of his *New Principles of Political Economy* he describes it as 'this astonishing country, which seems to be submitted to a great experiment for the instruction of the rest of the world'. Progress, rapid material progress, had become a fact. Observers were amazed at the profusion of wealth — 'a degree of wealth and luxury which surpasses all that can be seen in other nations'; they were amazed at the scale of manufacturing and commercial activity, the availability and speed of transport, the standards of comfort enjoyed, if not by all, at least by all above the ranks of manual labourer. In Manchester, or Glasgow, visitors found it impossible to contemplate 'the vast buildings and their dependencies' of modern industry without 'feelings of inexpressible astonishment'. In the central parts of London, convenience and magnificence combined to produce an atmosphere of luxury which would have seemed insolent if it had not been so respectable: 'that interminable succession of streets and squares, all consisting of well-built and well-furnished houses — the brilliancy of the shops — the crowd of well-equipped equipages'.[2] Early Victorian England, as G.M. Young put it, was a nation 'glowing with the authentic sense of war and victory'.[3]

This sense of triumph and of well-being was based essentially on the solid comfort of the well-to-do. But even for those less prosperous, down to the ranks of small farmers and skilled artisans, life was easier than before; the luxuries of the previous generation had become the necessities of this. The poor, of course, were as poor as ever, and there were probably more of them. Life had not been transformed in every respect. Poverty, pauperism, trade depression, riot and sedition; the 1820s and 1830s faced grave economic and political difficulties. Nevertheless, scientific progress and material progress continued and those who had already benefited from what one contemporary writer called 'the march of mind' could still hope that all problems, in due course, would be solved. Yet there was one problem that the early Victorians had not even begun to solve, one victory that they did not in the least look like winning: the victory (it can never be more than partial) over pain, and over sudden mortal illness associated with childbirth or with surgery.

In the hundred or so years before Queen Victoria ascended the throne, medicine, like other branches of science and technology, had not stood still. Indeed, one of its greatest practical triumphs had come in 1798, with the publication of Edward Jenner's *An Inquiry into the Causes and Effects of Variolae Vaccinae*. This small book, the result of many years of careful empirical work by a doctor in a country practice, showed convincingly not only that smallpox could be prevented by vaccination, but that its complete elimination by this means was feasible. Smallpox was one of the most dangerous of diseases, and was endemic in western Europe in the eighteenth century, outbreaks sometimes reaching epidemic proportions. The practice of vaccination, which as a result of Jenner's work now spread rapidly, must have had a considerable effect on the death rate, besides cutting down the incidence of serious illness and disfigurement. But aside from this signal instance of improved practice, medicine as it affected the vast majority of the population was not very different in 1840 from what it had been in 1740. Indeed, when John Stuart Mill expressed the hope, as late as 1861, that in times to come disease might be 'indefinitely reduced', he was relying primarily on 'good physical and moral education, and proper control of noxious influences', and only secondarily and in the more remote future on 'the progress of science'.[4]

Medicine was in a feeble state because medical education and medical research were at a low ebb. The quality of medical education in Britain in the first half of the nineteenth century was on average poor and in some respects deplorable. Generalisation is more than usually difficult, because a unified medical profession did not exist. Four distinct orders of medical practitioner could be discerned. There were pure physicians — socially, financially and by education at the head of the profession; pure surgeons, who were not expected to be men of superior education, and whose claim to be qualified, it was said, was that they were uncontaminated with the slightest knowledge of medicine; pure apothecaries, who could not be fully employed except in large towns; and doctors — apothecaries and surgeons in general practice who looked after the great bulk of the population.

Entry into each of these groups was by several methods which changed somewhat, and varied in importance, as time passed. Apprenticeship was by far the commonest road to qualification, especially in surgery, but in the second quarter of the century it was increasingly supplemented by instruction in private medical schools and teaching hospitals, and by 'walking the wards'. The whole system was casual and disorderly, the apprenticeship arrangements being subject to the usual abuses. Up to five hundred guineas might be paid as an apprenticeship fee to a fashionable doctor in London in the 1830s, but whether the fee was large or small, the doctor fashionable or otherwise, very little instruction was usually given; it was said that apprentices spent most of their time 'capping bottles and rolling pills', In England, the vast majority obtained a licence to practice — when they did obtain one, which was necessary only after 1815 — from the Society of Apothecaries; the other licensing bodies were the Royal College of Physicians and the College of Surgeons (which became the Royal College of Surgeons in 1843). The two Colleges dominated medicine in London until after 1850 and they were justly regarded as a sort of medical Oxford and Cambridge club; two universities where there was no adequate school of anatomy and no clinical hospital teaching. In Scotland, licences were issued by the four universities (five including Marischal College, Aberdeen), and by the Royal Colleges of Physicians and of Surgeons at Edinburgh and the Faculty of Physicians and Surgeons at Glasgow.

In the early decades of the century these numerous authorities made little or no attempt to co-ordinate their activities. They had a variety of rules for the students' attendance at lectures (frequently not given) and at hospitals, and a very large variety of fees. In the 1840s the usual course of study required four years (the apothecaries required a five years, apprenticeship) and no one could qualify under the age of twenty-one. The examination which the aspiring doctor had to pass, usually written and oral, might appear to be a genuine test of such knowledge as there was. But it was at this point that the really disastrous weaknesses of the system, if such it can be called, were to be found.

Most impartial observers agreed that the University of Edinburgh provided its students with the best organised and most thorough medical training to be had in Britain. In 1848 the final examination took 17½ hours and comprised twelve sections, preceded by two passages for translation from Celsus and from Gregory's *Conspectus Medicus*. The papers included the following questions:

(Chemistry) How is oxalic acid prepared? Give the formula both in the dry and in the hydrated state. Mention the best antidote to it when a poisonous dose has been given.

(Physiology) Describe the structure of the *medulla oblongata,* and state its functions, insofar as they appear to be known.

(Midwifery) State the diagnosis, the natural terminations, and the treatment of presentations of the shoulder.

(*Materia Medica*) State the principal characters of the elaterium plant, the nature, source, and preparation of elaterium, its proximate constitution, and its actions on the body.

(Practice of Physic) What are the essential articles of a truly tonic regimen?

(Natural History) State the general laws which regulate the trade winds, the monsoon winds, the sea and land breezes.

Fifty or so questions like these, to which was added the requirement of a small thesis (in Latin), gave reasonable opportunity for the student to reveal the extent of his knowledge, or for the examiners to uncover the extent of his ignorance. But as every teacher knows, the question in an examination decide nothing; however subtle or searching the questions, very paltry or absurd answers may be accepted for a pass. That this happened, even in Edinburgh, there can be little doubt. 'Many pass who are grossly ignorant',[5] it was said; and the 'grinders', who coached young men for the examinations frequently wrote their theses as well. Yet the average standard at Edinburgh was certainly higher than anywhere else. The courses of lectures were extensive and well-organised, the teachers were often men of outstanding ability and medical education was, in general, taken seriously.

Other schools aimed to do less and usually did much less. The best of them, University College, examined its students in only four divisions of medicine, for which lecture courses were provided. But in most cases the student was left to pick up what he could or what he thought suitable by reading, going to a few lectures, and listening to what was said and watching what was done in a hospital. The years required for this 'instruction' — usually four — had to be filled in somehow, and were apt to be spent in 'idleness and sensual gratification'; medical students had an unenviable reputation for drunkenness and debauchery. When the examination approached, the typical student took himself off to a grinder, who gave the necessary preparation in 'three weeks of questions and answers by rote'. The examinations were commonly referred to as a farce; in the 1820s the Apothecaries' Hall conducted an annual examination compared with which, it was declared, 'that in the farce of Molière ceases to be a caricature'.[6] Similar terms were used to describe the ways of examiners at the Royal College of Surgeons 30 years later:

> . . . the momentous question whether a third-year's student was fit to practice surgery upon Her Majesty's subjects was decided off-hand, after dinner, in one hour's time, by four ancient surgeons, who 'tackled' the young gentlemen for a quarter of an hour each successively, and propounded various anatomical and surgical conundrums for his entertainment. If the candidate's powers of endurance lasted out the hour he duly passed . . . without having had his anatomical knowledge tested on the dead subject, or his surgical acumen on a living patient. *Mutatis mutandis,* the same farce was enacted at the Apothecaries' Hall . . .[7]

Even as late as 1868 Syme declared that medical education was

> a preparation . . . merely for passing examinations which, for the most part, imply neither an accurate knowledge of facts nor the possession of sound principles, being simply affairs of memory loaded with dry terminology.[8]

And to make matters worse favouritism and nepotism were rife, certainly in the Royal Colleges.

Low standards, apathy and neglect were not confined to London or to England. In 1841 the examination for MD at St Andrews consisted, apart from the usual Latin translation, of 102 questions of which the first six and the final five were as follows:

> Where is the heart situated?
> In what mediastinum?
> How many cavities has it?
> What are they named?
> What are the vessels leading out of it?
> How many?
> What are the diseases of arteries?
> What are the consequences of ossification of arteries of the brain?
> What do you understand by an aneurism?
> What operations are performed for the cure of aneurism?
> What is the most approved treatment for varicose veins?

Nine candidates sat this examination. One failed and eight passed, all between ten o'clock in the morning and four o'clock in the afternoon. Such proceedings were not untypical of British medical education in the 1840s. No wonder that in 1844 a gentleman wrote to the *Lancet* saying that one of his sons 'directly he became an MRCS, went on the continent, and visited and studied at most of the continental schools and hospitals, including Edinburgh and Dublin', and that he now wished that his youngest son should 'get through his studies by the time he is one or two and twenty, that he may then *seek knowledge* in some of the continental schools. . .'[9]

The English approach to medicine in the first half of the nineteenth century — and to a much lesser extent the Scottish approach also — combined an almost medieval respect for tradition with an excessive admiration for the manners and attainments of an eighteenth-century gentleman. There was something in it of the cloister, and something of the club. Thus an Edinburgh graduate could appeal confidently to his fellow doctors not only because, like him, they had a working knowledge of the limited range of drugs in use and of the old-fashioned, complicated prescriptions, but because they too were men who could be relied on

in point of classical and medical education, scientific tastes and acquirements, sound physiological and pathological views, and the manners and feelings of gentlemen of cultivated minds.[10]

Sometimes the emphasis on the classics seemed overdone, even to contemporaries. In the College of Physicians, according to one writer to the *Lancet,*

> classical attainments are made of greater importance than in either the Law or the Church. Candidates for the licence, looking forward to the fellowship, think more of passing a good classical, than a sound medical, examination. Scanty physiology and pathology, decked out in respectable Latin, will stand higher than mere professional excellence, marred by a false concord, or a fault of prosody.[11]

But the system possessed an advantage which the profession very well understood; they knew that this kind of learning 'kept up their reputation with the public'; people in all walks of life, profoundly ignorant of medicine, were aware that doctors were men of superior education and, on this basis, went on to give them credit also for being skilful physicians.

As long as medical science was in a rudimentary state there was something to be said for the old attitude; we know that the physiology and pathology which these doctors half learnt was not much use anyhow. By the 1840s the physical and natural sciences had made a lot of progress, but medicine had not kept up. As the *Lancet* put it, 'the information of the medical profession, generally, on matters of natural science, is very little greater than that of the people at large. This is an extremely humiliating fact.'[12] And this was increasingly important, because science had come to affect medical understanding at several points: for example, it was a simple and direct application of chemistry to diagnosis that had established the connection between granular disease of the kidney and albuminous urine. In these circumstances, pressure to apply to medical problems the techniques and findings of physical and natural science was bound to increase, and was quite noticeable by the later 1840s. This led to a struggle between the new attitudes of scientific observation, experiment, reasoning and innovation, and old attitudes of classical culture and conservatism. And this struggle between the new science and the old learning was the general background to the controversies over anaesthesia and, even as late as the 1870s, antisepsis.

But the practice of medicine was only gradually affected by new scientific ideas and scientific ways of thinking; after all, the leading members of the profession in the 1830s had received their education in the eighteenth century and few of those who were most prominent in the 1870s had graduated later than 1840. Most doctors before 1850, and many as late as 1870, it would seem, simply did not observe or think scientifically; one wonders sometimes if many of them thought at all. Thus in the 1830s one member of the profession reported the discovery that a cause of epilepsy was indulgence in venery; six out of seven recent cases that had come his way, he reported, 'were decidedly owing to venereal excitement'. In one case the health of a patient aged 41 'was completely re-established by a voyage to America, leaving his wife in England'; in another, that of a young man of 23 who evidently (the language of the report is very guarded about this) masturbated, 'the only mode of treatment that was adopted was counter-irritation to the part affected. A diet consisting principally of fish and farinacious food, with constant employment in business from morning till night . . . before the expiration of six weeks thoroughly established his health'.[13] Eight years later a series of articles appeared in the *Lancet* on 'the law of seven', seeking to show that seven was a magic number in medicine: 'whatever type the fever may exhibit, there will be a paroxysm on the seventh day . . . and . . . the fourteenth will be remarkable as a day of amendment' — and concluding, after several thousand words, with 'the question of lunar influence'.[14] There is no reason to suppose that readers of the most progressive medical journal in England found these articles absurd or out of place. And as it was with the profession so, inevitably, it was with the public. In 1855 Syme, Professor of Clinical Surgery at Edinburgh, reported

the case of a lady from London, whom I was asked to see a few days ago. On visiting her, I was asked to pay special attention to the spinal processes of two of the lumbar vertebrae, which it was said were too far apart. I could find nothing wrong, and my informant — the lady's husband — had some difficulty in pointing out the situation of the supposed affection, which I, however, explained could be of no earthly consequence even if it did exist. The gentleman then, assuming a very serious aspect, asked this question: supposing the bones to be a little too far apart, would this allow the sinovial fluid to escape from the joints of the spine, and descend along the back, so as to form an ovarian tumour in the pelvis? I need not say that a person capable of repeating such preposterous nonsense would not be in a fit state to accept any information on the subject consistent with common sense. Yet these were people of high consideration and great intelligence, and possessing the means of access to the best sources of information.[15]

This is typical Syme — accurate and forthright. But Syme himself was anything but typical, and most of the profession wallowed in careless observation, slovenly thinking, and ancient habits.

Of these last, bleeding was probably the most widespread. Doctors had bled their patients for hundreds of years in season and out of season, and they continued to do so well into the nineteenth century. When in 1850 Sir Robert Peel fell from his horse and suffered concussion, a comminuted fracture of the left clavicle, a fractured rib, and internal haemorrhage, from which injuries he shortly died, he was attended by the best doctors in London. Thirty hours after the accident 20 leeches were applied. But many members of the profession thought that he should have been 'bled to a large amount'. The antiphlogistic system of treatment, taught in all medical schools in the 1830s and 1840s, recommended copious bleeding, violent purgatives, and poor liquid diet for almost every kind of illness or malfunction. Liston, in 1835, complained about 'the disgraceful scenes which I have more than once witnessed, of bleeding patients almost *in articulo,* and on the brink of the grave. . .'[16] But it might be almost as bad to be given a prescription. Acetate or superacetate of lead combined with opium was prescribed for haemorrhage of the lungs; a prize fighter suffering from dimness of sight, loss of movement, and 'an appearance of idiotcy' was given (at St George's) purgatives, calomel, opium and strychnine; acne rosacea was successfully treated with up to twenty minims of kreosote given internally three times a day — the patient developed a variety of disturbing symptoms, but recovered; Liston knew a patient in Edinburgh who 'had been treated to no less than six courses of mercury for gonorrhoea . . . his health was now quite broken. . . He had ulcerated palate to a fearful extent, abscess in the corner of his eye . . . and there was such a discharge and such foetor as were quite overpowering. It was almost impossible to come within arm's length of him.'[17] No wonder that the fatal termination of many illnesses was attributable to the doctor rather than to the disease.

Ignorance of the action of drugs only partly explains this frightful state of affairs. There was also the fact that careful physical examination of the patient was unusual in the 1830s and none too common before 1850. In urging 'sedulous examination . . . regardless of the time required', an exceptionally enlightened physician in 1826 wrote as follows:

> I have known a female patient, labouring under obstruction of the bowels, with evident symptoms of inflammation, on being question-ed whether there was any swelling about the groin, or whether she had ever been subject to rupture, deny the fact; yet the surgeon, confident that the urgent symptoms . . . could not take place with-out adequate cause, urged the necessity of examination, and, on its being reluctantly submitted to, immediately discovered a small femoral hernia.[18]

Most doctors were content to enquire about previous illnesses and present appetite, to feel the pulse, and to observe the appearance of the eyes, tongue, urine and faeces, in that order of interest. Because they seldom attended to or even looked for local symptoms and abnormali-ties they were apt to be content with prescribing 'a farrago of stuff from a *vade mecum*' in the hope that this would influence the patient's general condition. It was indeed easier to prescribe than to think. The *Lancet* blamed 'the old ladies at Rhubarb Hall' (i.e. the apothecaries) who had 'done all that in them lay to convert the medical practitioners of this realm into pill-mongers',[19] but the apothecaries probably met rather than created the demand. The truth was, that the doctors simply did not know enough about medicine. And it was this that brought homeopathy into vogue. Giving only minute doses, insufficient to affect the patient's health one way or the other, the homeopathists, whether they knew it or not, depended on 'the expectant principle' which says that a little coloured water, taken with the assurance that it is a powerful emetic, will produce vomiting. In the circumstances, homeopathy was often a great deal better than orthodox medicine; it at least gave an opportunity for spontaneous recovery. In the middle decades of the century the doctors railed constantly against 'the foul waters of quackery', which, they said, raged like a torrent, and in which they included homeopathy. But homeopathy was often to be preferred to 'the drugging principle', which was the essence of approved British practice.

Doctors faced other difficulties besides a wholly inadequate know-ledge of pathology, and of drugs. Those who favoured physical examin-ation of the patient, for example, lacked the elementary tools to carry it out. The stethoscope was invented in the eighteenth century, but it found little favour in Britain before the reign of Queen Victoria. This was because few doctors learnt how to use it. Many hoped, on its introduction, that it would forthwith 'unveil the morbid mysteries of nature . . . to the crude perceptions of the merest tyro in the profession'; when this did not happen the stethoscope was very generally laid aside. It was much the same with the thermometer. Instruments of this kind existed; but they were so large that contemporaries compared them with umbrellas; and in any case they took about 20 minutes to register. On the other hand, an increasing amount of work was being done in morbid anatomy (the Anatomy Act of 1832 made bodies legally available for dissection) and this encouraged the practice of clinical examination, because examination of the patient became much more revealing when it could be related back to what had already been found, in other cases, in the post-mortem room. In pathology also there were fresh beginnings. Johannes Müller, who has been described as possibly the greatest physiologist of all time, made outstanding contributions to the physiology of the nervous system, beginning in the 1830s, and his path-breaking work on tumours was based on the novel and enormously important idea of the cell as a functional unit. For much of his research he depended on the use of the microscope, and in this respect also he was a pioneer.

These and other developments were important, and they were all potentially of very great importance. But their immediate impact was often small. As late as the 1860s, for example, the upper social reaches of medicine — which were not necessarily the highest technical reaches — were still largely governed by the practices of the previous century. Physicians to the Royal Family at that time seem seldom to have taken anyone's temperature, never refer to examination of urine for albumen or sugar, and did not always time a patient's pulse. Quinine was 'the sovereign remedy', being exhibited for almost everything from orbital neuralgia to nervous exhaustion. 'The only drugs used which had real effects were opium and aperients.'[20] In 1872 Sir Henry Holland, who had 'set up an all-time record by attending no less than six Prime Ministers of England, not to speak of two English Queens, a Prince who became the Emperor Napoleon III, as well as four leading poets — and did all this without really being interested in medicine, as his *Memoirs* make abundantly clear'[21] — took the view that the prescription, 'however learned in its Latin and pharmacy', was of much less consequence than 'watchfulness over the economy of the sick chamber . . . all, too, that the *lenis sermo* and *hilaris vultus* (I willingly quote from Celsus) can justifiably do in soothing and giving hope'.[22] This is not altogether foolish, but it seriously underestimates the importance, or at least the potential importance, of scientific and technical medicine.

Fashionable doctors may have been abnormally out of date, and in any event their patients were few. What affected the lives of vastly more people and drew a great deal of attention in the second quarter of the nineteenth century was the campaign to improve public health. Asiatic cholera reached Britain from the East for the first time in 1831, and in the following two years deaths from this cause totalled over 30,000. An outbreak of cholera was a spectacular disaster, and it was doubly important because it affected rich and poor alike; 'it struck terror into the minds of the middle and upper classes',[23] and hence led to some administrative reform. Such reform, unhappily, was as a rule short-lived, because whereas cholera came and went, administrative reform was troublesome to initiate and even more troublesome to maintain. In any case what killed people in substantial numbers year after year was not cholera but typhus and consumption. These diseases killed especially in the towns. And as more and more of the population came to live in the overcrowded and insanitary slums of the early-to-middle nineteenth century, typhus and consumption became more and more prevalent. Concern over the general health of the urban population emerged in the 1830s and reached new levels in the 1840s; and by the end of that decade the public health movement was born. Medical opinion from the 1780s had increasingly underlined the connection between insanitary, overcrowded conditions and disease. (Typhus, remarked one writer in the 1830s, 'might not inaptly be termed the poor man's disease')[24]. Therefore the obvious move was to improve the water supply, improve (or more often provide) sewerage, and put an end to the practice of building as many dwellings as possible, every one of them as cheaply as possible, on every urban acre.

These measures gradually took effect. But little of all this can be connected with the advance of medicine, because the process of the diffusion of disease continued to be misunderstood or not understood at all. Until the time of Lister, the doctrine that prevailed was that of Galen — his doctrine or a debased version of it. Galen taught that the cause of epidemics was atmospheric corruption acting on bodies already predisposed to disease. This atmospheric corruption might arise from 'a multitude of unburned corpses as may happen in war; or the exhalations of marshes and ponds in the summer; sometimes it is immoderate heat of the air itself as in the pestilence which Thucydides describes'. But the victim had to be, so to speak, in a receptive condition:

No cause can be sufficient without an aptitude of the body; otherwise all who are exposed to the summer sun, move about more than they should, drink wine, grow angry, grieve, would fall into a fever.

The most likely 'aptitude of the body', according to Galen, was malnutrition.

This 'theory' has a very Greek sound about it. The basic idea is that nature acts upon man, but man also acts upon himself. The 'causes' which arise in nature and help to produce disease, are necessary but not sufficient. This explanation was plausible in the sense that it was consistent with most observations. Moreover, the Greeks did not ignore the obvious facts of contagion and infection. They recognised that those attending the sick often caught the disease themselves, and that articles used or handled by sick persons and then passed on to others seemed to spread infection. But they regarded these facts as relatively unimportant.

The authoritative work on this subject in the early nineteenth century was *A Treatise on Fever*, written by Southwood Smith and published in 1830. Southwood Smith, who was a dissenter, had taken his medical degree at Edinburgh in 1816, and in the same year had published *Illustrations of the Divine Government*, a work of which the sixth edition appeared in 1866. In his *Treatise* he argued that poverty resulted from ill health, especially from the ravages of epidemic fever; and he subsequently played a very important role in the public health movement. Southwood Smith may fairly be called an advanced thinker; but a few sentences from his book will show how Galen's doctrine continued after 1600 years almost without alteration:

The immediate, or the exciting cause of fever is a poison formed by the corruption or the decomposition of organic matter. Vegetable and animal matter, during the process of putrefaction, give off a principle, or give origin to a new compound, which, when applied to the human body, produces the phenomena constituting fever.[25]

The room of a fever-patient, in a small and heated apartment of London, with no perflation of fresh air, is perfectly analogous to a stagnant pool in Ethiopia, full of the bodies of dead locusts. The poison generated in both cases is the same; the difference is merely in the degree of its potency. Nature, with her burning sun, her stilled and pent-up wind, her stagnant and teeming marsh, manufactures plague on a large and fearful scale: poverty in her hut, covered with her rags, surrounded with her filth, striving with all her might, to keep out the pure air, and to increase the heat, imitates Nature but too successfully; the process and the product are the same, but the only difference is in the magnitude of the result. Penury and ignorance can thus at any time, and in any place, create a mortal plague.[26]

This was what came to be called the miasmatic theory of disease, and in the hands of some writers it was reduced to the simple proposition that bad smells breed diseases. This of course was wrong. But those who laboured in the middle decades of the century to get rid of dunghills in towns, and bad sanitation, and impure water supply, and overcrowding, were working in the right direction. They showed good sense; although it cannot be said that they possessed good science.

Thus although medicine made advances and took part in others in the early nineteenth century, it was clearly not in the van of progress; and were a present-day patient suffering from (let us say) scarlet fever or anaemia, to find himself alive in that departed world, his experience would be, to say the least of it, a very unpleasant one and possibly quite short. But what would be unrecognisable — totally, horribly unrecognisable — would be the experience of a surgical patient who was transported back to the world of the 1830s. Surgery, like medicine, had not stood still during the eighteenth century and the early nineteenth century. A more thorough knowledge of normal and pathological anatomy was now at the command of a good surgeon, he had more and better instruments than his predecessors, and operations were now being performed, sometimes with success, that would not have been attempted a century before. Yet the early Victorian surgeon had much more in common with the barber surgeon who marched with the army in the campaigns of Marlborough than with his successors today.

In the first place, the surgeon, unlike the physician, had the misfortune to be obliged to do most of his work in hospital. In many cases, if the patient could afford it, he was operated on in his own home; but most people were not so lucky. The best that can be said of the hospitals of the early nineteenth century is that those of the preceding century were often worse. It is small praise. True, a number of old hospitals had recently been rebuilt, or new wards or theatres had been added. For example, a new anatomical theatre and museum were built at St Thomas's in 1813, several additions and enlargements were made at St Bartholomew's between 1822 and 1854, and a surgical wing was added to the old Edinburgh Royal Infirmary (the foundation stone of which had been laid in 1738) in 1829.[27] Moreover, the management of hospitals began to be affected by what the eighteenth century called 'the fresh air regimen' and by the idea that dirt and disease were somehow connected. Notice began to be taken of such elementary principles of hospital hygiene as the opening of windows, as well as (though this was less common) the washing or disposal of dirty or infected articles and the sweeping of floors. The isolation of fever patients also became more common; Edinburgh, for example, opened a separate fever hospital in 1818. In view of the fact that 27.9 per cent of all deaths in England and Wales in the last six months of 1837 were due to diseases of respiratory organs,[28] measures of this kind were clearly important.

But, on the whole, hospitals, even the best hospitals, remained dark and overcrowded, ill-run and insanitary. It was not uncommon to see in the same ward, at the same time, cases of, (let us say) typhoid fever, erysipelas, pneumonia, rickets, dysentery; nor was it uncommon to see two patients in the same bed — perhaps a man with a broken leg alongside a patient in the last stages of consumption. (A guide book to Edinburgh published in 1825 stated with pride: 'In this hospital [Royal Infirmary] the male and female patients are kept entirely distinct; and 228 sick people can be accommodated in separate beds'.[29] The consequence was that many patients who were admitted to hospital with one complaint soon contracted another, with possibly fatal consequences. Washing facilities were very poor, and in many cases were not accessible to the patients.[30] The nursing staff were for the most part taken off the streets; women who were uneducated, unskilled, poor, slovenly, and often more interested in alcohol than in their patients. Not surprisingly, it was a common complaint that food and medicine supplied for one patient found their way to another — or to no patient at all. Above all, the hospitals stank. John Howard, who did so much for prison reform, recorded in 1789 that the wards of the hospitals he visited 'were often so offensive as to create the necessity of perfuming them; and yet I observed that the physician, in going his rounds, was obliged to keep his handkerchief to his nose'. Well over half a century later, the situation was little different. Sir Hector Cameron was Lister's house-surgeon in Glasgow in the 1860s, and in later life he recalled how 'every surgical ward, no matter how well ventilated' was filled with 'a foetid, sickening odour, which tried the student on his first introduction to surgical work just as much as the unaccustomed sight of the operating theatre'.[31]

The typical operating theatre of the first half of the nineteenth century would strike a modern observer with the utmost astonishment. The words 'operating theatre' are indeed somewhat euphemistic, for what they described was often only a moderate-sized room, which, apart from its size, in some ways resembled a market place rather than an operating theatre. It was apt to be ill-lit and, according to one surgeon who had seen these rooms as a young man, 'grimed with the filth of decades'. There were no masks, no gloves, no sterilising vessels of any kind. The surgeon himself might wear a suit, having removed the jacket and possibly rolled up his sleeves. By the 1850s it was more common to wear a special 'surgical coat'.

> When a dresser or a house-surgeon entered upon his term of office he hunted up an old coat, in the lapel of which he probably carried a wisp of ordinary whipcord for tying arteries. This garment did duty for six months or a year, and was then very properly discarded. There was no such time limit, however, for the surgeons themselves. Their operating coats lasted from year to year, and eventually acquired an incrustation of filth of which the owners appeared unconscious, or even proud.[32]

If the weather was cold, there might be a fire burning in an open fireplace. The floor would be plain, unpolished deal, sprinkled with sawdust around the operating table. Close by the table would be chairs for colleagues and distinguished strangers, and, a little further back in a teaching hospital, any number of students; all dressed in their ordinary, workaday clothes. There would also be an instrument clerk nearby, seated at a small table. If the operation was exceptional, so was the number of spectators: theatres were sometimes 'crowded to the door'. In 1831 it was reported that the operating room at St Bartholomew's was 'last Saturday . . . so crowded that scarcely one half of the pupils could see what was going on, and after uselessly endeavouring for some time to remove the obstruction by crying out "Heads, etc" ' they sent down a paper of complaint. But the patients had more reason to be concerned than the students.

> Should anything occur during an operation not exactly looked for or expected, or should the surgeon ask for any instrument or thing not in the hands of the house-surgeon, great interruption must of necessity occur, [the house-surgeon] having of necessity to force his way backwards and forwards through the crowd.[33]

In such unassuming and, so to speak, homely circumstances, in which there was little sense of preparation or precaution, a patient might find that an operation had been carried out almost before he was aware of it. In 1861 a student of Syme's recorded the case of

> an old surly-looking fellow, who was brought in, suffering from a very rare disease north of the Tweed, viz. Chimney Sweeper's Cancer on Scrotum. When asked by Professor Syme if he had ever been south of the Tweed, he said in a very surly tone, 'Aye, I hae been to Perth'. 'Had he ever swept chimneys?' 'Na!' When asked if he would take chloroform or not, he made no reply. Professor Syme with a pair of scissors at once cut out the cancer which was situated on the most dependent part of the scrotum. The shouts of the old fellow were terrific. Professor Syme, after he had completed the tying of the vessel cut, questioned him concerning the period of its growth, and got for a reply: 'Hoo the devil can I answer any questions just noo?' This created a very hearty laugh among the students, which did not improve the temper of the patient. He left the theatre uttering imprecations on Professor Symne and all concerned.[34]

But it was not often that what happened in an operating theatre gave rise to laughter. Except to those accustomed to it, the mere sight of a nineteenth-century operation before anaesthesia was a ghastly experience. To newcomers, it was frequently unbearable. When Charles Darwin was a student of medicine at Edinburgh in 1828, he 'attended on two occasions the operating theatre . . . and saw two bad operations, one on a child, but I rushed away before they were completed. Nor did I ever attend again, for hardly any inducement could have been strong enough to make me do so; this being long before the blessed days of chloroform. The two cases fairly haunted me for many a long year.'[35] Simpson himself had a similar experience when he was a student. He went on one occasion to see Robert Liston, one of the two or three greatest surgeons of the day, carry out an operation for amputation of the breast. The technique 'was to lift up the soft tissues by an instrument resembling a bill hook, enabling the surgeon to sweep round the mass with his knife, in two clean cuts'. As the operation began, Simpson fled. 'He turned away, pushed through the crowd of young men and left the room. He hurried out of the hospital gate and up the hill to Parliament Square, where he burst into the imposing building and asked where he could work as a clerk, declaring in an agitated voice that he wanted to study law.'[36] Fortunately for humanity, the following day he changed his mind.

In the modern world, at least in the West, pain is mitigated and death is kept discreetly out of sight. Our forefathers were vastly more familiar with both, and pain, like death, was accepted as a condition of life. It was as a rule borne with fortitude, and the Victorians were inclined to regard its endurance without complaint as a virtue: 'a young wife would say to the midwife after her first confinement, "I didn't flinch, did I? Oh, I do hope I didn't flinch." '[37] What went on in an operating theatre, however, was an entirely different matter. The most hardened observer and the most resolute patient might well give way before the ordeal. Dragged unwillingly or carried from the ward to the operating theatre by a couple of hospital attendants (in Edinburgh a large wicker basker was used for this purpose) the patient was laid on the operating table and if necessary strapped down, surrounded by curious strangers. The first cut of the scalpel must have caused searing pain, and few patients were able to clench their teeth and remain silent. Shriek after shriek were more likely to fill the room, ebbing away to convulsive cries and sobs as the operation proceeded. Finally, prostrate with pain and exhausted by the calculated violence that had been used, the patient was carried back to the ward from which he or she had come only a short time before. No wonder that Lister once referred to surgery as 'this bloody and butcherly department of the healing art'.

From the earliest days physicians had been searching for means to relieve pain in surgery. Alcohol was an obvious possibility, and wine and brandy were frequently used for this purpose, necessarily on the day of the operation.[38] Medieval doctors favoured a 'sleeping sponge' or 'soporific sponge', saturated with drugs such as opium or mandragora; and this method was still sometimes used in the early nineteenth century. This meant, of course, application not through the mouth but by inhalation. Mesmerism was tried, usually unsuccessfully (a Scots doctor working for the East India Company had good results in Bengal, but on his return to Scotland found his own countrymen less susceptible to hypnosis); compression of the nerves to the site of the operation was another idea that had a brief vogue; while French surgeons were inclined to prefer bleeding the patient to the point of insensibility. All these methods were partially or in some cases totally ineffective, and had serious disadvantages of their own. They were peculiarly unsuitable for women in childbirth, but this was not seen as important because pain in childbirth was regarded as 'natural', the inevitable and indeed the proper lot of womankind. There was also the idea that the agonies of child-birth were the effect of a little understood variety of disease. In any case, relieving this form of pain was not an accepted medical objective.

Pain in surgery being thus regrettably unavoidable, what the surgeon aimed to do was to limit its duration as far as possible. He had to work fast. Many operations, it is said, were measured in seconds, and if a student looked away for more than a moment he might find that he had missed just what he had come to see. Liston, whose course of lectures at Edinburgh Simpson attended, was noted for speed, and Simpson admired him for it; he operated 'with such speed', Simpson wrote, 'that the sound of sawing seemed to succeed immediately the first flash of the knife'. Thus in his *Remarks on the Operation of Lithotomy* Liston observed that, 'should there be but one or two stones of a moderate size (under the size of a hen's egg), the incision and extraction should not occupy more than two or three minutes at most'.[39] A thorough knowledge of anatomy, enormous confidence, speed, resource, dexterity – these, and sometimes strength, were what a good surgeon needed. In some operations Liston was exceptionally successful because of the strength of his fingers and his muscular power. In amputation of the thigh, for example, he sometimes dispensed with a tourniquet and instead compressed the femoral artery with one hand while he removed the limb with the other. This was, in a sense, brilliant surgery; but its scope could not be too ambitious. Complicated operations, which took time to perform, were out of the question; they had been followed too often by disaster. Hence abdominal surgery was not often attempted. In Ballingall's *Outlines of Military Surgery*, published in 1833, it is stated that:

> Wounds of the small intestines are for the most part either primarily or secondarily fatal . . . No man in his senses would think of enlarging the external wounds, for the purpose of searching out and sewing up the wounded part of the gut. . . It must ever be recollected that bleeding from the arm is the best preservative from internal bleeding and peritoneal inflammation. . .[40]

Even so, some surgeons were bolder than others, and ovariotomy – the removal of a cyst on the ovary – was becoming commoner in the 1850s. Why it was not more common may be deduced from the following description of one of the first operations of this kind, performed by Ephraim McDowell in Kentucky in 1809:

> Having placed her on a table of the ordinary height, on her back, and removed all her dressing which might in any way impede the opera-

tion, I made an incision about three inches from the musculus rectus abdominis on the left side continuing the same nine inches in length . . . extending into the cavity of the abdomen. . . The tumour then appeared full in view, but was so large that we could not take it away entire . . . We took out fifteen pounds of a dirty gelatinous-looking substance, after which we cut through the Fallopian tube and extracted the sack, which weighed seven pounds and one half. As soon as the external opening was made, the intestines rushed out upon the table; and so completely was the abdomen filled by the tumour, that they could not be replaced during the operation which was terminated in about twenty-five minutes.[41]

There was no anaesthestic. The patient survived, and lived for another thirty years. She was, to say the least of it, lucky as well as courageous; even the most skilful and experienced operators in the 1850s and 1860s had to be content with a death rate from ovariotomy in the region of 50 per cent or over. Operations on the spinal column and the cranial cavity were even more difficult and dangerous, and were correspondingly even less common.

If so much of the human body was beyond the reach of surgery, what, it may well be asked, kept the surgeons employed? A good deal of their work arose from wounds of all kinds, and compound fractures; and operations for the treatment of aneurism were not uncommon. But the striking difference between the practice of surgery before and after about 1850 — for anaesthesia made a difference here — is that in the earlier period amputations were an everyday affair; they were, so to speak, the staple diet of surgery. In the early 1860s, at St Bartholomew's, 21 per cent of the operations were amputations, and at University College in the later 1860s the proportion was rather over 25 per cent. These percentages are perhaps a hundred times larger than would be shown by present-day figures, yet they are certainly smaller than the percentages that prevailed in the first half of the century. Then, long and complicated operations to repair a damaged joint or limb were not attempted, not necessarily because the surgeon was not skilful enough but because, in the absence of anaesthetics, the patient would probably die of shock and exhaustion: in many cases of even slight injury to a wrist or elbow joint 'there will be great risk attending a simple resection, owing to the extensive suppurations which will inevitably occur around the wound . . . it will be safer to amputate'.[42] Injured hands or legs that were already suppurating badly had to be removed. In an enormous number of cases amputation was the only remedy.

That surgeons concentrated on a limited range of operations, and that speed was essential, does not mean, therefore, that most operations were in any sense 'minor'. On the contrary, a very large percentage of operations were life and death affairs because no one in his senses would submit to an operation except as a last resort; the patient was frequently almost beyond help before he arrived in the operating theatre, and the surgeon might therefore be compelled to adopt heroic measures. Major surgery, within the limits possible, was consequently not uncommon, and it placed an appalling strain on the surgeon as well as the patient. 'The human being placed under the surgeon's care and submitting to the trial upon his advice, was sure to skirt the borders of death, and would in a few minutes after he had placed himself under the knife, quivering and conscious . . . moan, grow pale and yet paler, with white lips and beaded brow, until the grey of death perhaps crept into the blanched face.'[43] Few surgeons can have enjoyed their work. Hunter, for example, spoke of operating as an unavoidable evil; Cheselden is said always to have turned pale when about to cut for the stone; Sir Charles Bell, whose dexterity and coolness as an operator were remarkable, was often seen to blanch as he proceeded with operations carried out with the utmost self-possession and skill; Sir Spencer Wells the pioneer leading ovariotomist of the mid-nineteenth century, commented that in the days before chloroform surgeons like himself 'had to nerve themselves up to the infliction of the most deliberate and tedious eviscerative vivisection'.

Those who carried out such operations had to work beyond the range of ordinary emotions, and many of them were men of remarkable ability and character. The greatest British surgeons of the period were almost certainly Liston, Fergusson and Syme. All were Scotsmen, and all were graduates of Edinburgh University. Liston, after a brief spell in London, taught anatomy in Edinburgh alongside Syme for several years and then, when Syme was appointed to the Edinburgh Chair of Surgery in 1833, returned to London and became Professor of Clinical Surgery at University College in 1835. Although not a scientific surgeon — he made few original contributions to surgery — he was a brilliant operator, and strength and dexterity, coupled to a surpassing knowledge of anatomy, enabled him to carry out feats of surgery which, for speed and resolution, have probably never been and never will be surpassed. He carried out the first surgical operation in Britain using anaesthesia, and died less than a year later, at the age of 53. Ferguson was born in 1808, fourteen years after Liston and became a

Fellow of the Royal College of Surgeons in Edinburgh when he was only 21. By the mid-thirties he and Syme were the most successful surgeons in Scotland. In 1840 Fergusson was appointed Professor of Surgery at King's College, and he rapidly became the leading operator in London, where he 'astonished the world by his marvellous feats of surgery'. He was distinguished not only as a very successful professional man — he became surgeon to the Prince Consort and later to the Queen — but also as the first great exponent of 'conservative surgery', a phrase first used by him in 1852. All parts of the body were to him sufficiently important to try to save, and he revived and improved upon many operations for this purpose, as well as devising new ones. His contribution to the advance of surgery was in this way very important. He also impressed contemporaries by his self-command and cool temper, and by the 'exceeding care' with which his operations were prepared for, and conducted.

Syme, like Liston, was by date of birth a man of the eighteenth century, although only just; he was born in 1799. He began the study of anatomy under Liston at the age of 19, and in 1833 became Professor of Clinical Surgery at Edinburgh. By the middle of the nineteenth century he was at the height of his powers, a great teacher and a great practical operator; 'the first of British surgeons', wrote Lister, when he met him in 1852. There was nothing ostentatious about Syme's speech, his manner, or his style of operating, yet his personality as well as his mastery of his profession immediately and deeply impressed everyone who came in contact with him. Merely to see him operate was for many a revelation:

The merest tyro sees at once a master of his craft at work — no show, little elegance, but absolute certainty, ease and determination . . . the patient is sent off, still anaesthetised, and then comes a brief commentary, short, sharp, and decisive, worth taking down verbatim if you can manage it; yet he has no notes, a very little veiled voice, and no eloquence.[44]

When still in his early twenties, Syme had demonstrated his powers in an extraordinary way. As a young man of 24, while lecturing on anatomy at Edinburgh, he had successfully performed an amputation through the hip-joint for the first time in Scotland. This operation, in his day 'the greatest and bloodiest in surgery', Syme had never before assisted at or even seen. But he carried it out under the eyes of his seniors with a confidence born of a thorough knowledge of anatomy, surpassing technical skill, and an iron nerve. His composure in an operating theatre never left him; he never raised his voice. Yet through the years he was responsible for 'feats that were probably the most hazardous that any one man has dared, and dared successfully, upon the living bodies of other men'.[45]

But Syme was much more than a remarkable operator. He was also a man of ideas. Many new operations which he devised, and many of his other contributions to surgical practice, have become classics in the art of surgery. Also, he took part, often with decisive effect, in several of the great medical controversies of his time. He was a man of strong and firmly-held opinions, and he was never afraid to say what he thought. His prejudices, according to those who disagreed with him, were neither few nor small, and in some ways this may have been true; but he had a capacity for logical thought probably unique among the surgeons of his generation.

Hunter, Cheselden, Bell and Liston were all great surgeons; but in their day no surgeon, however great, could have much confidence in the final outcome of his work. He knew, only too well, that after even a simple operation carried out in a technically flawless manner, the patient carried back to the ward might be dead in a week. The early-nineteenth-century surgeon was like a medieval peasant (it was a surgeon who said so), who, having sown the seed, could only wait with resignation to see what it might please Almighty God that the harvest should bring.

The trouble was that no one understood or could control the process of the healing of surgical wounds. This process may take place, as the nineteenth century put it, either 'by first intention', that is to say, without inflammation or suppuration; or 'by second intention', that is, through the gradual filling of the cavity with a rudimentary form of tissue called granulations, the process being a prolonged one, accompanied by more or less inflammation and suppuration and probably fever. Until Lister had done his work, healing by first intention was scarcely expected, save after operations on certain parts of the body, such as the face. Healing by second intention was the rule. In this latter case, if all went well, post-operational suppuration, inflammation and fever were not prolonged. The flow of pus from the openings provided for drainage gradually diminished after the first week or two, the wound became less inflamed, the fever subsided, and after several weeks or even months, the patient recovered. Surgeons were well satisfied with such a result, 'and were full of self-congratulations if anything better was achieved'.[46]

In the mid-nineteenth century surgeons spoke of four septic diseases — so-called 'hospital diseases'. These were erysipelas, pyaemia, septicaemia, and hospital gangrene. Before the 1860s or 1870s surgeons did not at all clearly distinguish one of these diseases from another. Erysipelas varies in intensity, from an angry blush on parts of the face, to extensive inflammation and suppuration among the muscles. Pyaemia is characterised by the formation of septic clots in the veins, which clots, or parts of them, travel along the blood stream to the lungs and other parts of the body, giving rise to abscesses. Septicaemia included several conditions, but meant, on the whole, blood-poisoning in which clotting in the veins was absent or unimportant. Hospital gangrene was a process of mortification which turned living tissue into a moist grey slough, surrounded by an angry blush, and was progressive. These were all forms of sepsis, and in each case there took place the formation and spread of pus within the body.

Surgeons watched the onset and development of these diseases with anxious and usually despondent care:

Though you expect to procure adhesion, or at least to make some part of the wound adhere, you are often disappointed; you are sensible, from the violence of the fever and the swelling of the limb, that mischief is going on within. The dry skin, the parched mouth, the thumping pulse, the restlessness and delirium, continue for some days, and there is a blackness round the wound threatening gangrene. But this fever by degrees becomes less violent, the livor, which proceeded partly from ecchymosis [spread of blood beneath the skin], partly from the dark colour of the inflammation, gradually changes to green, the great wound begins to suppurate and open very wide, the whole limb swells to an enormous degree, the skin and cellular substance are soft and relaxed, and bear the impression of the finger, the redness extends all over the limb, and from the particular hollowness and softness of certain points you are sensible that great suppurations are forming within.

All your prudence, and more especially all your diligence, is required for conducting this stage of the disease. . . You are careful to dress the limb every morning, and perhaps to clean it also a little in the evening. By regular washing and wiping with the moist sponge, you prevent those smells which depress the patient's spirits, and injure his health; and by laying clean lint to the wounds twice a-day, you soak up the foul matter. . . How much is due to care and cleanliness, you may judge from this, that in the case of a gentleman who lies in his own house, we often venture to save a limb, which, had the accident befallen a poor man lying in a crowded hospital, must have been cut off. . .

Often it happens, from the destruction of parts, or the unhappy circumstances of the patient, that all your cares are unavailing! every time you examine the limb, you make discoveries of more extensive destruction, you find the whole limb swelling every day more and more, you find the matter running profusely from the openings, the openings increasing in number and the suppurations extending from the ham to the heel with intolerable foertor, the muscles all undermined, and the bones carious. You find that you are no longer able to support the patient's health, that repeated attacks of diarrhoea and fever have reduced him to extreme weakness; and the wan visage, the pale and flabby flesh, the hollow eyes and prominent cheekbones, the staring and squalid hair, the long bony fingers and crooked nails, the quick, short breathing, and small piping voice, declare the last stage of hectic and debility! the natural powers are then sunk so low, the appetite for food, and even the desire of life so entirely gone, that we would believe the patient past all help, did we not know by experience that it is never almost too late to amputate the limb.[47]

These terrible, painful, and commonly fatal illnesses − 'the pain is dreadful; the cries of the sufferers are the same in the night as in the day-time; they are exhausted in the course of a week, and die: or if they survive, and the ulcers continue to eat down and disjoin the muscles, the great vessels are at last exposed and eroded, and they bleed to death'[48] − these illnesses were liable to ensue in almost any surgical case, indeed, in any case where the skin was cut or even bruised. This was what made the situation peculiarly dreadful. A patient suffering no more than a compound fracture (that is, a broken bone with the skin torn either by the force of the injury or by the bone itself) might find himself within a week with all the symptoms of gangrene and signs of approaching death. 'In hospitals, especially in military hospitals, and most of all in hospital-ships (which the Lords of the Admiralty would do well to burn), the patient sinks almost inevitably under the suppuration of a compound fracture.'[49] These words were written at the very start of the nineteenth century; but 50 years later the position was not, in essentials, any different. Even a scratch might lead to a septic condition and prove mortal: many such cases are recorded. Of the forms of sepsis, hospital gangrene was the most dangerous and uncontrollable. Bell's dramatic advice regarding this disease has often been quoted:

> Let [the surgeon] bear this always in mind, that no dressings have ever been found to stop this ulcer; that no quantities of wine or bark which a man can bear, have ever retarded this gangrene; let him bear in mind, that this is a hospital disease; that without the circle of the infected walls the men are safe; let him, therefore, hurry them out of this house of death . . . let him lay them in a school-room, a church, on a dunghill, or in a stable . . . let him carry them anywhere but to their graves.[50]

But sepsis did not occur in all cases. Some wounds surgical as well, as accidental, healed 'naturally' without complication, and in many cases without medical assistance of any kind. It was also observed that in simple fractures, in which the skin was not broken, healing took place without suppuration or obvious inflammation, however severe or extensive the injury below the skin might be. The obvious conclusion was, that when the skin was broken something entered or might very likely enter the wound which gave rise, in some unexplained way, to sepsis. And the further obvious conclusion was drawn that this something was the air. But perhaps not all air. In the latter half of the eighteenth century doctors and surgeons noted with increasing frequency the apparent connection between dirt and disease, and between 'foul air' and disease. This observation was the foundation of the public health movement, already mentioned; and within the hospitals it was the justification of efforts towards greater cleanliness and more fresh air. But these efforts were half-hearted, partly because of conservatism and inertia, partly because, in almost any surroundings, some wounds healed without difficulty whereas others did not, partly because surgeons believed — and it seemed not unreasonable — that direct attention to and management of the wound was bound to have more effect than the establishment of favourable general conditions. Accordingly, the principal efforts of surgeons continued to be devoted to excluding air from the wound or, alternatively, to counteracting, in whatever way seemed best to the surgeon concerned, its malign influence.

Excluding the air — the so-called 'occlusion method' — was attempted by covering the wound with collodian, goldbeater's skin, caoutchouc, and even adhesive plaster. If in these circumstances suppuration never began, all was well; but if it did begin the consequences were almost sure to be disastrous, because the poison, unable to escape, transmitted its full force into the patient's blood stream. When Syme was a young surgeon in the 1820s, this was the method he found most used in Edinburgh. He soon gave it up, however, in favour of immediate stitching of the wound, with openings left for drainage, and the application of what was (fondly) supposed to be a dry dressing. This method was taken over by Lister when he, in his turn, was a young surgeon at Edinburgh in the 1850s, and was later described by him in the following words:

> This [method] consisted of points of interrupted suture at sufficient distance from each other to afford a free outlet for discharges, and pads of folded lint applied over the bodies of the flaps but not extending to the lips of the wound, with a broad piece of lint over all, and a bandage applied so as to press the deep surfaces of the wound gently together through the medium of the pads; while the cutaneous margins were left free for the exit of the discharge, which was absorbed by the lint as it escaped. This dressing was left undisturbed for about four days, when union was found already pretty firm; and a similar application being afterwards repeated at intervals of two days, the discharge of pus was commonly very trifling in amount, and the cure speedily accomplished.[51]

But success was by no means certain; even Lister, before he devised antiseptic surgery, lost patients using this method. Other surgeons favoured occlusion with repeated opening, a policy described and denounced by Liston in the 1840s:

> Wounds . . . are put together without delay, and their edges having been squeezed into opposition are retained so by various means, such as sutures, plasters, compresses, and bandages. They are carefully covered up and concealed from view for a certain number of days. Then the envelopes of cotton and flannel, the compress cloths, the pledgets of 'healing ointment', as it is called, and plasters are taken away, loaded with putrid exhalations, and a profusion of bloody, ill-digested, foetid matter. A basin is forthwith held under the injured part, and the exposed and tender surface is deluged with water from a sponge, not always over-clean, and then well squeezed and wiped. Then comes a reapplication of retentive bandage, of the plaster, of the grease. . . The process is repeated day after day; the patient is kept in a state of constant excitement, and often, worn out by suffering, discharge, and hectic fever, falls a victim to the practice.[52]

Liston himself was an exponent of what was called 'water-dressing'. This meant joining the surfaces with sutures of waxed silk or fine wire, and then applying bandages soaked in water. These were supposed to keep the wound cool. If suppuration set in, the sutures were removed, and a large soft linseed poultice was applied, usually as hot as could be borne. (In at least one London hospital, according to Godlee, the poultice was the most commonly used dressing well into the 'eighties of the last century'.) Another treatment, favoured by some, was frequent or continuous irrigation; sometimes the affected part, or even the whole patient, was immersed in water which was constantly being changed. This method was soothing to inflamed wounds, and in other cases was at any rate not a cause of actual irritation. Moreover, it was markedly successful in preventing the onset of septic disease, which is not surprising, for, unlike all others, it assisted the removal of discharges as soon as they were formed. But it was cumbersome and expensive, was declared to be in some cases 'unnecessary or really injurious',[53] and was more common in German than in British hospitals.[54] Controversy raged as to whether the water should be hot, tepid, or cold. Those who favoured the last could go one step further, and apply ice. Used constantly and freely', this was claimed to be particularly effective in preventing the spread of inflammation.

The variety of treatments, of which the above is a mere summary, shows how surgeons struggled desperately and confusedly to control post-surgical inflammation, suppuration, and fever. Patients might be seriously ill for one or two weeks, or for any period of time up to, say, six months; and then they might recover, or they might die. Why some recovered, and why some died, no one really knew. Even more important, no one knew why and how they became ill in the first place. It was agreed by an increasing number of doctors that the trouble was probably caused by pollution of the atmosphere; but what this pollution might consist of was not in the least understood, and the mechanism was totally unexplained. Nevertheless dirt and overcrowding seemed to make matters worse, and a number of surgeons responded in a perfectly sensible way. In 1862 one of them described his practice in the following words:

The local treatment may be summed up in two words — repose and cleanliness. The cleanliness should, however, include more than it commonly does, such as the use of general or large local baths, the value of which . . . cannot be overstated; and of the frequent change, not only of dressings, if there be any, and of bed-linen, but of beds. . . As to general treatment, the best plan is to let the patient be as ready as possible in the ordinary mode of prudent life, to give no medicine of which the need is not expressly indicated, to observe all rules of personal cleanliness, to provide abundant fresh air, and a sufficient or a liberal mixed diet.[55]

This passage is notable, not only for its display of common sense, but also for emphasising that cleanliness, to be effective, had to be more thorough-going than was often understood. Much that was common practice in hospitals was deplorably unhygienic. In 1862, for example, it was thought worth saying that 'the bandages and instruments which have been employed for gangrenous wounds ought not, if possible, to be employed a second time; nor should bandages, linen, or clothing, be prepared or kept in rooms where infected patients are lying'.[56] And there was also the question how fresh had fresh air to be? Were there, perhaps, varieties of fresh air? From Germany came a report that 'in many desperate cases of these diseases, where every means had been employed in vain, and the patients seemed past hope, an immediate change for the better was perceived' when they were taken into the garden 'and left for the rest of the day under the nice foliage of the beautiful plantains'. But was improvement due to the fresh air, or the plantains? No one knew. The German comment was that it was best if the patient could be placed 'under foliage, the exhalations from which are well known to have a very beneficial effect'.[57]

It is not possible to say much about the causes and rate of mortality after operations. These must have varied a great deal from time to time, mortality reaching appalling levels when, for example, wards were invaded by hospital gangrene, and almost equally from place to place, for one surgeon who was a believer in genuine cleanliness might accomplish much. And the figures themselves are not very revealing. Many a patient died not as a result of the operation but because the operation failed to arrest the course of the disease from which he or she suffered. This was often so with hernia, tracheotomy and trephining. Patients also suffered from such mysterious post-operational maladies as 'icteric irritative fever' and 'acute sinking'. In other cases patients died from readily identifiable diseases which 'fall, as it were, casually on those who have been operated on'. Typhus and scarlet fever were diseases put in this category; but it could be asked, of course, whether the surgeon was not responsible for averting this sort of 'casual' misfortune. Nineteenth century statistics took no notice of these difficulties, and one has only crude figures of post-operational mortality. At University College Hospital, even in the early 1870s, the rate of mortality after amputation was stated by the then Professor of Clinical Surgery, Sir John Erichsen, as lying between 24 and 26 per cent, and this he thought 'may be regarded as somewhat satisfactory'.[58] This was in the light of figures (presumably comparable) of 39 per cent at Glasgow, 43 per cent at Edinburgh, 46 per cent at Zurich (1860–7), and 59 per cent at Paris (1836–63). Another figure, relating to 1859, and not limited to amputations, shows a post-operational death rate of 28 per cent.

How many deaths occurred in or as a result of child-birth is equally hard to determine. The principal danger in this case was the onset of puerperal fever a few days after delivery. There is some evidence that the greater provision of lying-in hospitals in the first half of the nineteenth century increased the incidence of the disease, and this is more than likely. But no one can be sure, if only because physicians were entirely uncertain about the nature and symptoms of the illness. They were equally unsure about its treatment. Was it an inflammatory disease, or was it quite distinct from peritonitis? Would it bear bleeding, or was the smallest loss of blood inadmissable? On such fundamental questions there was no agreement. The doctors were united on only one point; puerperal fever was apt to spread and they did not know how to stop it: 'The obstetrician who meets with one case may generally expect others, no care that he can take being sufficient to prevent the infection from spreading.'[59] In the 1840s an increasing number of doctors were not only asking themselves how puerperal fever spread, but also why it sometimes occurred after an apparently safe and easy confinement. The answers to these questions were not generally known in Britain before 1850, but Simpson was one of those who understood that surgical fever and puerperal fever had many characteristics in common. As early as 1840 Simpson was teaching his students that puerperal fever was a disease communicated from one patient to another by the doctor or midwife going from one case to the next. But what the material was, Simpson could not explain. He noted, like several others, that lack of cleanliness and of fresh air seemed to promote the disease, and he began the campaign for smaller, airier, less crowded wards: 'if our present medical, surgical and obstetric hospitals were changed from being crowded places, with a layer of sick in each flat, into villages or cottages, with . . . at most two patients in each room, a great saving of human life would be effected'.[60] But to implement such a proposal would have cost an enormous sum, and in any case many doctors remained unpersuaded that puerperal fever was not transmitted directly from one patient to another. All that was certain was that many women died from this cause. In the 1840s it was reckoned that 3,000 mothers died from puerperal fever every year in England and Wales. If correct, this meant a death rate, from this cause alone, of approximately one in every 210 confinements. This is certainly possible, because in the 14 months to the end of 1870 the Edinburgh Royal Maternity Hospital, recently re-opened with all modern sanitary improvements, showed a maternal death rate of 1 in 223, which was claimed to be the best in the United Kingdom. The figure for the whole of London at that time was reported to be 1 in 190.

## Notes

1. J. Priestley, *Essay on Government (1768)*, p.6.
2. Quoted in G.M. Young, *Early Victorian England,* vol. I (Oxford, 1934), p.171.
3. Ibid., vol. II, p. 418.
4. J.S. Mill, *Utilitarianism,* (Everyman edition), p. 14.
5. *Lancet,* vol. II, (1848), p.327.
6. *Lancet,* vol. I, (1825–6), p.4.
7. *Lancet,* vol. II, (1872), p.476.
8. *British Medical Journal,* vol. I, (1868), p.371.
9. *Lancet,* vol. I, (1844), p. 302.
10. *Lancet,* vol. II, (1848), p.81.
11. *Lancet,* vol. I, (1847), p.38.
12. *Lancet,* vol. I, (1842–3), p.127.
13. *Lancet,* vol. II, (1834–5), p.13.
14. *Lancet,* vol. I, (1842–3), p.127.
15. *Lancet,* vol. I, (1855), p.398.
16. *Lancet,* vol. I, (1834–5), p.549.
17. *Lancet,* vol. I, (1834–5), p.549.
18. *Lancet,* vol. I, (1825–6), p.217.
19. *Lancet,* vol. I, (1842–3), p.686.
20. N.M. Goodman, 'Medical attendance on Royalty', in F.N.L. Poynter (ed.), *Medicine and Science in the 1860s* (London, 1968), p.134. The above paragraph is based almost entirely on Dr Goodman's excellent and entertaining chapter.
21. Ibid., p. 135.
22. Ibid.
23. M.W. Flinn, Introduction to Edwin Chadwick's *Report on the Sanitary Condition of the Labouring Population of Great Britain* (Edinburgh, 1965), p.10.
24. R. Miller, *Clinical Lectures* (Glasgow, 1833), p.11, quoted in Flinn, ibid., p.10.
25. Southwood Smith, *A Treatise on Fever* (London, 830), pp.348–9.
26. Ibid., p. 364.
27. This wing was not a new building. It was the old High School which had been built in 1777.
28. Stated in *First Annual Report on the Registrar General* (1839), pp.166.
29. J. Stark, *Picture of Edinburgh* (Edinburgh, 1825), p.242.
30. In Edinburgh there were 'hot and cold baths . . . and other baths are

appropriated for the citizens at large', in J. Stark, *Picture of Edinburgh*, p.242.

31. Quoted in G.T. Wrench, *Lord Lister, His Life and Work* (London, 1913), pp.66–7.

32. R.J. Godlee, *Lord Lister* (Oxford, 1924), p.129.

33. *Lancet*, vol. II, (1831–2), pp.31.

34. Quoted in Myrtle Simpson, *Simpson the Obstetrician* (London, 1972),

35. T.H. Huxley, 'Charles Darwin', in G. de Beer (ed.), *Autobiographies* (Oxford, 1974), pp.25–6.

36. M. Simpson, *Simpson the Obstetrician*, p.41.

37. F. Thompson, *Lark Rise to Candleford* (Penguin, 1973), p.50.

38. A sailor who had his thigh amputated without an anaesthetic during the Crimean War was asked about the pain. He replied that it had not been severe, 'for you see, Sir, they gave me the best part of a bottle of rum before they began, and I didn't find much of it'. *Lancet*, vol. II, (1872), p.521.

39. *Edinburgh Medical and Surgical Journal*, (January, 1825), p.26.

40. G. Ballingall, *Military Surgery* (London, 1833), p.539.

41. McDowell's account as given in Harvey Graham, *Eternal Eve* (London, 1950), p.423.

42. *Year Book of Medicine, Surgery, and their Allied Sciences for 1862* (London, 1863), p.196.

43. Wrench, *Lord Lister*, p. 40.

44. Dr Joseph Bell, one of Syme's house-surgeons, quoted in J.D. Comrie, *History of Scottish Medicine*, vol. II (London, 1932), p.599.

45. Wrench, *Lord Lister*, p.40.

46. Godlee, *Lord Lister*, p.145.

47. John Bell, *The Principles of Surgery*, vol. I (Edinburgh, 1801), pp.655–8.

48. Bell, *The Principles of Surgery*, p.110.

49. Bell, *The Principles of Surgery*, p.657.

50. Bell, *The Principles of Surgery*, p.117.

51. In T. Holmes's *A System of Surgery*, 2nd edn (Edinburgh, 1871), vol. V, p.614.

52. R. Liston, *Practical Surgery*, 4th edn (London, 1846), p.31.

53. *Year Book*, (1862), p.190.

54. In Germany at one time there were 'wards containing rows of large baths in which patients with running sores lie supported on sheets, eating and sleeping, day and night, and apparently enjoying themselves like fishes in a stream'. Godlee, *Lord Lister*, p.152.

55. *Year Book*, (1862), pp.178–9.

56. *Year Book*, (1862), p.213.

57. *Year Book*, (1862), p.213.

58. *Lancet*, vol. I, (1874), p.85.

59. *Lancet*, vol. I, (1842–3), p.879.

60. See *Edinburgh Monthly Journal of Medical Science*, vol. IX, (November, 1848), pp.329 ff.

# 2　THE ADVANCE OF ANAESTHESIA

The discovery of inhalation anaesthesia belongs to the extensive category of 'multiple discoveries', that is to say, discoveries made not once by a single person but at much the same time and in much the same form by several persons working quite independently. It is also an example of a discovery made not solely by 'the discoverer' but dependent to a substantial extent on information and ideas supplied by predecessors and contemporaries. It is true that in the case of inhalation anaesthesia the build-up of knowledge and experience reached, after a time, a critical point; there was a day – 16 October 1846, to be precise when inhalation anaesthesia was first used with success by a surgeon in an operating theatre in the presence of expert witnesses. That day marked a great step forward – one of the greatest that has ever been taken – in the reduction of human suffering. But at the same time it should be seen as another stage in a long process of discovery and development that had already gone on for over a century and was to continue to the present day.

It is not difficult to follow the chain of discovery back to the later seventeenth century. In 1667 Robert Hooke, Professor of Geometry, physicist, architect, demonstrated before the Royal Society that the movement of the lungs was not, as was commonly supposed, requisite for the circulation of the blood, but was needed in order to keep an adequate supply of fresh air in contact with the lung tissue. A little over a hundred years later Joseph Priestley liberated the gas which we call oxygen, and noted not only that 'a candle burned in this air [oxygen] with a remarkably vigorous flame', but also (in 1775) that a mouse could survive longer in oxygen than in an equal volume of 'common air'. At almost exactly the same time, on the other side of the Channel, Lavoisier was carrying out research on combustion and on the respiratory process. Aided by Priestley's results, he was able to show that air consists of two elastic fluids, one of them – 'the most salubrious part of the air' – essential for respiration and combustion, the other non-respirable and incapable of supporting combustion. Continuing his work into the 1780s, Lavoisier showed, in collaboration with Laplace, that oxygen was changed into carbonic acid in the process of respiration, and he argued that it was to this process that animal heat is due:

Respiration is then a combustion, admittedly very slow, but never-theless completely analogous to that of charcoal; it takes place in the interior of the lungs, without liberation of perceptible light, because this matter of fire [a supposed element that Lavoisier believed to be present in air] is no sooner liberated than it is ab-sorbed by the humidity of these organs. The heat which is produced in the combustion is transmitted to the blood which passes through the lungs and from thence it courses through the whole animal system.

In 1789, five years before he was led to the guillotine, Lavoisier further showed that while respiration is the same in any concentration of oxy-gen, as long as carbon dioxide is removed, the amount of oxygen ab-sorbed varies with temperature, food and work load.

These brilliant researches carried understanding of the respiratory process to new levels, and gave rise to the idea that different 'kinds' of air might be useful in combating disease. Priestley, who agreed with many of his contemporaries in believing that carbon dioxide could check putrefaction, first suggested that the gas might with benefit be inhaled:

Being satisfied that fixed air [carbon dioxide] is not noxious *per se* . . . I hinted to some physicians of eminence among my acquain-tance, that it may possibly be of use in the case of ulcerated lungs, if persons in that most deplorable situation would breathe as much as they found they could do of it, by holding their heads over vessels containing fermented mixtures. . . Those gentlemen were pleased to think favourably of the proposal, and I am informed by Dr Percival[1] that the same ideas had occurred to other persons, and that in three cases in which the breathing of fixed air had been tried, it appeared to have been of great service. One patient intirely recovered. . .[2]

Other gases were tried. Priestley himself inhaled oxygen in 1775, and although he did not suggest that it might have therapeutic value − his comment was, 'who can tell but that, in time, this pure air may become a fashionable article in luxury. Hitherto only two mice and myself have had the privilege of breathing it' − inhalation of oxygen, especially in cases of asphyxia, soon become established in medical practice. In 1796 it was reported from Birmingham that 'the vapour of vitriolic aether' [sulphuric ether] was being inhaled by patients suffering from phthisis pulmonalis, with 'the best effects':

The first effects of this application are an agreeable sensation of coolness in the chest, an abatement of the dyspnoea and cough, and, after ten minutes or a quarter of an hour, easier expectoration . . . The only unpleasant circumstance attending the inhalation of this aethereal tincture of cicuta [ether containing extract of hemlock] is a slight degree of sickness and giddiness, which, however, soon go off. . .[3]

Pneumatic medicine, as these forms of treatment came to be called, was by the end of the century at the height of its popularity.

Its greatest proponent was Thomas Beddoes. After studying medicine at Oxford, Beddoes became Reader in Chemistry at that University and published, about 1791, two small volumes entitled *A Letter to Erasmus Darwin, MD, on a New method of treating pulmonary consumption and some other diseases hitherto found incurable* and *Observations on the nature and cure of calculus,*[4] *sea scurvey, consumption catarrh and fever.* These publications aroused much interest, and Beddoes was led on, with the help of some friends, to establish an institution for research into the use of gases in the treatment of disease and into the best methods of preparing and applying them. This institute, with apparatus designed by no less a person than James Watt, was begun in Bristol in 1794, and was called the Pneumatic Institution. Its achievements in the way expected of it were small. But it provided in one vital respect a link in the chain of discovery, for in the autumn of 1798 Beddoes appointed Humphry Davy, at the age of nineteen, to be Superintendent of the new institution. (Davy's first contact — a very indirect one — with pneumatic medicine took place in 1797, when a friend of Beddoes encountered him 'idly swinging on a half-gate' outside the house of the Cornish surgeon to whom young Davy was apprenticed. Beddoes first met Davy in the summer of 1798, while on holiday in Cornwall. He did not offer him employment on the spot, but the appointment was arranged within a few months. However mistaken his belief in the curative properties of gases, Beddoes must have had a keen eye for native ability.) Using the laboratory facilities thus placed at his disposal, Davy continued and extended investigations which he had already begun in Cornwall into the properties of nitrous oxide. His experiments included inhalation of the gas, and he found that this produced 'a sensation analogous to gentle pressure on all the muscles, attended by an highly pleasurable thrilling . . . [but] whenever its operation was carried to the highest extent, the pleasurable thrilling . . . gradually diminished . . . impressions ceased to be perceived; vivid ideas

passed rapidly through the mind, and voluntary power was altogether
destroyed, so that the mouthpiece generally dropt from my unclosed
lips'.[5] Nor did Davy fail to note that inhalation of nitrous oxide could
reduce the sensation of pain, without producing unconsciousness:

> The power of the immediate operation of the gas in reducing intense
> physical pain, I had a very good opportunity of ascertaining.

> In cutting one of the unlucky teeth called dentes sapientiae I ex-
> perienced an intense inflammation of the gum, accompanied with
> great pain which equally destroyed the power of repose, and of con-
> sistent action.

> On the day when the inflammation was most troublesome, I breathed
> three large doses of nitrous oxide. The pain always diminished after
> the first four or five inspirations, the thrilling came on as usual, and
> uneasiness was for a few minutes swallowed up in pleasure. As the
> former state of mind, however, returned, the state of the organ
> returned with it; and I once imagined that the pain was more severe
> after the experiment than before.[6]

That the pain increased after and by inference as a result of the inhalation was of course an illusion. But this mistake did not prevent Davy
from suggesting that nitrous oxide might find a place in surgery:

> As nitrous oxide in its extensive operation appears capable of des-
> troying physical pain, it may probably be used with advantage dur-
> ing surgical operations in which no great effusion of blood takes
> place.[7]

These words were written in 1800, and for a moment science stood on
the verge of a great discovery. Indeed, a great discovery had been made,
if anyone had recognised it. But no one did. Even Davy himself does
not seem to have attached importance to the idea, which he tucked
along with several other concluding observations at the end of his
book; and of course his advocacy of nitrous oxide as an analgesic was
severely qualified by his reference to 'no great effusion of blood'. These
words may reflect Davy's belief that nitrous oxide increases the force of
the circulation of the blood, and would therefore make the control of
haemorrhage more difficult.[8] Also, this reservation is a vague one, and
would seem to rule out anything except very minor surgery. So perhaps

it is understandable that no one followed up the suggestion. As for Davy himself, he concluded that pneumatic medicine could make no progress until numerous fundamental physiological and chemical relations were established, and more experience gained. In 1801 he resigned from the Institution, and never again attended to medical problems.

Pneumatic medicine survived, but it made little progress. Clinical experiments in inhalation continued but produced no very significant or valuable results. Instead, the problem of anaesthesia in relation to surgery was clearly stated, and solved after a fashion, by a young doctor in Shropshire, working on his own quite outside the mainstream of speculation and experiment; what he wrote and suggested, however, was completely ignored. His name was Henry Hill Hickman. He was a member of the Royal College of Surgeons in England and of the Royal Medical Society of Edinburgh, and in 1823, at the age of 23, he conducted a series of experiments in which dogs, mice and rabbits were placed in a confined space and compelled to reinhale their own breath (or carbon dioxide introduced into the chamber) until they lost consciousness; Hickman then operated upon them 'without the slightest appearance of pain'. The animals recovered, and the wounds healed. Hickman was well aware of the significance of this work. In 1824 he wrote to T.A. Knight, a Fellow of the Royal Society who lived nearby and was possibly an acquaintance, explaining that:

> From the many experiments on suspended animation I have won-dered that some hint has not been thrown out, of its probable utility, and noticed by Surgeons, and, consequently, I have been induced to make experiments on Animals, endeavouring to ascertain the practicability of such treatment on the human subject, and by particular attention to each individual experiment I have witnessed results which show that it may be applied to the animal world, and ultimately I think will be found used with perfect safety and success in surgical operations.[9]

A few months later Hickman published a pamphlet entitled *A Letter on Suspended Animation, containing experiments showing that it may be safely employed during Operation on Animals, with the view of ascertaining its probable utility in surgical operations on the Human Subject.* This pamphlet was 'addressed to T.A. Knight Esq', and in it Hickman expressed the hope 'that you will think the results sufficiently interesting to induce you to do me the honour to lay them before the Royal

Society'. Nothing came of this, and in 1828 Hickman went to Paris and tried to interest Charles X of France. In this also he failed (although his letter was passed on to the *Académic Royale de Médicine*) and two years later he died.

Why was this remarkable initiative unsuccessful? No doubt its very novelty was against it. Moreover, the idea that patients should first be partially asphyxiated and then operated on is somehow unappealing – it savours more of violence than of medical care; and as for inhaling carbon dioxide, that might not be safe. Hickman was careful to point out that 'I have never known a Case of a person dying after inhaling Carbonic Acid Gas, if proper means were taken to restore the animal powers', and in writing to Charles X he spoke of inducing insensibility 'by means of the introduction of certain gases into the lungs'; what these 'certain gases' were, however, he did not specify. But the principal difficulty was probably Hickman's isolation. He tried to attract the attention of the Royal Society, which was an entirely sensible thing to do, but the Society did not respond, or else remained unaware of his approach. He might, one fancies, have tried the Royal Medical Society of Edinburgh, of which he was, after all, a member; but he may have realised that at this period the Edinburgh medical school was in a weak state, suffering from, among other ailments, inbreeding and nepotism. Beddoes, whom Hickman probably knew of, had died in 1808. Sir Humphrey Davy was alive, but by 1824 his health was failing and he looked back on his time at the Pneumatic Institution as 'misemployed'. To have appealed to any of the leading surgeons of the day would almost certainly have been useless; surgeons were craftsmen, or perhaps in a dreadful way artists; they were certainly not experimental scientists, and their training gave them very little knowledge indeed of this kind of activity. Today, a man in Hickman's position would write to some appropriate journal, describing his work and outlining his ideas. But in the 1820s this was scarcely possible. The *Lancet* was begun only in 1823, and in 1824 Hickman may very well never have seen or heard of it. *The British Medical Journal* first appeared in 1857, its lineal predecessor in 1853. *Nature* was founded in 1869. When he tried the Royal Society, Hickman probably did the best he could.

Further progress came by a very different route. At the Pneumatic Institution both Beddoes and Davy entertained visitors and no doubt impressed them by giving them an opportunity to inhale nitrous oxide. Most people enjoyed it. Robert Southey, for example, found it 'a sensation perfectly new and delightful' and S.T. Coleridge, who had experience in these matters, recorded 'an highly pleasurable sensation' and added that 'the only motion that I felt inclined to make was that of laughing at those who were looking at me'. Others danced, jumped about, or rolled on the floor. One elderly gentleman of a gloomy disposition had the good fortune to find that the effects were permanent; after inhaling three quarts of the gas his gloomy disposition left him, 'and has given place to an uniform cheerfulness'.[10] It was widely agreed that an alternative to champagne had been discovered, and inhaling nitrous oxide − or alternatively ether vapour; it was soon noticed that the results were the same − gradually became a slightly fashionable amusement, not confined to students of chemistry.

Ether frolics and nitrous oxide parties seem to have been commoner in the United States than in Great Britain, and in the former country it also became a practice for itinerant lecturers, possibly possessing not much more than an inflatable bag and an elementary knowledge of chemistry, to travel round the country giving demonstrations of the effects of 'laughing gas' − it was usually ether, because ether was easier to obtain, store and administer − and offering their audience an opportunity to try it. Such is not, as a rule, the stuff of scientific advance. But it was from these by no means serious activities, in which many of the participants engaged only, as would be said nowadays, 'for kicks', that in the brief space of two years inhalation anaesthesia was born.

There was, perhaps, an abortive preliminary. In 1852 a young doctor named Crawford Long, working in Georgia, stated that ten years previously he had come to realise, after taking part in 'ether frolics', that bruises or injuries sustained by those under the influence of ether were not at the time noticed to be painful, and that this had led him to believe 'that anaesthesia was produced by the inhalation of ether, and that its use would be applicable in surgical operations'.[11] He had, according to his account, carried out three small surgical operations in 1842 using ether, without any evidence of suffering being caused to the patients; and had carried out several more in subsequent years. These events, if they took place, were the start of surgery using inhalation anaesthesia; but they led to nothing. Unlike Hickman, Long made no attempt to spread the news of his discovery, or to persuade others of the importance of what he had done. No one outside Georgia, perhaps no one outside Long's practice, knew anything of the matter until the revelation of 1852. It seems strange. Surely there were other doctors in Georgia whom Long knew and met occasionally, and who would have been glad − and whose patients would have been still more glad − to know of the possibility of painless surgery. Long claimed that he proceeded cautiously, that he was not sure that his cases were representative, that his opportunities for experiment were limited. But this defence is not very convincing. If he had an idea of such great potential importance and lacked the means to test and develop it, he should have handed it on to others who could do so; on the other hand, his failure to do this must raise a doubt whether he himself realised the importance of the idea. In any event, the fact remains that what he did was of no consequence for medical history.

In 1844, however, a Boston dentist called William Morton become interested in anaesthesia. Unlike Long, Morton was ambitious, possessed considerable determination, and, as events were to show, was of an avaricious cast of mind. Secretive, calculating, and devoid of any unusual store of scientific knowledge, Morton appears as neither a great nor a particularly likeable man. Nevertheless, it was he, along with his one-time partner, Horace Wells, who bridged the gap between the use of ether as an idle entertainment and its first successful application in surgery.

At the end of 1844 Wells attended an exhibition 'of the effects produced by inhaling Nitrous Oxide, Exhilarating or Laughing Gas' put on in Hartford, Connecticut, by an itinerant lecturer called Colton who had at one time studied medicine but had never taken a degree. This exhibition, according to the handbill that advertised it, was to be 'scientific to those who make it scientific'. It also promised some fun:

Eight Strong Men are engaged to occupy the front seats to protect those under the influence of the Gas from injuring themselves or others. This course is adopted that no apprehension of danger may be entertained. Probably no one will attempt to fight.

The effect of the Gas is to make those who inhale it either Laugh, Sing, Dance, Speak or Fight, and so forth, according to the leading trait of their character . . . NB The Gas will be administered only to gentlemen of the first respectability. The object is to make the entertainment in every respect a genteel affair.

In the course of the evening it was noticed, as it had been noticed by Long, that injuries sustained by those staggering about and falling down under the influence of nitrous oxide were not accompanied by any feeling of pain; and it occurred to Wells that if nitrous oxide were administered to a dental patient, painless extraction might be possible. Apparently on the spur of the moment, Wells, having 'a wisdom tooth that troubled him exceedingly', went to his office, accompanied by the itinerant Colton and his bag of gas, and there inhaled the gas and then had his tooth extracted by another dentist. The experiment was successful. 'A new era in tooth-pulling!' Wells exclaimed.

He did not underestimate the importance of what he had discovered. Within a month he had carried out 15 painless extractions, and then, evidently realising the possible scope of inhalation anaesthesia, he went to Boston in the hope that he could attract the attention of the surgeons at the Massachusetts General Hospital. He approached his old partner Morton, who introduced Wells to a couple of surgeons at the hospital, who expressed interest. It was arranged that Wells would give a demonstration of extraction with anaesthesia before physicians and students. This demonstration took place but was only partially successful, probably because insufficient gas was given — Wells's apparatus was exceedingly elementary and his experience was limited. Several of the audience 'expressed their opinion that it was a humbug affair', and on this single trial Wells was rejected in the leading centre of medicine in the United States. The next day, deeply discouraged, he returned to Hartford.

But Morton, who had been present at Wells's demonstration, was not so easily convinced that inhalation anaesthesia in surgery was an impossible dream. Morton had already used liquid ether as a local anaesthetic on a sensitive tooth; he knew, as many others did, that the vapour of ether mixed with air could just as well as nitrous oxide produce partial or complete insensibility; and being in his practice much concerned with the removal of broken tooth stumps before fitting dental plates (not all dentists followed this procedure) he was particularly concerned to alleviate the pain thus caused and, as a result, to enlarge his practice. In 1846 Morton began experimenting upon animals, and from this he went on to try the effects of ether first upon himself, then upon two of his assistants, and then upon a patient 'suffering under the most violent toothache'. The ether was inhaled from a saturated handkerchief, and the patient 'did not experience the slightest pain whatever'. Attempts to repeat this success, however, resulted in failure; and Morton, all the time working as far as possible in secret, turned to a local instrument maker for some more manageable device for administering ether. He was supplied with a tabulated glass globe receiver into which was put a piece of sponge, to be kept saturated with ether. One opening to the retort was to admit air into the interior of the globe, while through the other vapour was to be drawn into the lungs. This inhaler was soon improved by the provision of a leather flap valve, hung so as to open during inspiration and close during expiration; this replaced the simpler but far less satisfactory arrangement of having the patient breathe to and fro into a valveless but not quite closed flask. Breathing was entirely oral, the patient's nostrils being held closed by the administrator or his assistant.

Before these improvements to the inhaler were complete, Morton approached John Collins Warren, senior surgeon at the Massachusetts General Hospital, and offered to demonstrate his new method of inhalation anaesthesia. Warren, although he had had to do with the Wells fiasco the year before, expressed interest. And on 16 October 1846, Morton brought the latest (and untried) version of the inhaler to the General Hospital and proceeded to anaesthetise a young man of 20 suffering from a tumour on the neck. Warren was the surgeon, and the following is his description of this famous occasion.

> The patient was arranged for the operation in a sitting posture, and everything made ready. . . The patient was then made to inhale a fluid from a tube connected with a glass globe. After four or five minutes he appeared to be asleep, and was thought by Dr Morton to be in a condition for the operation. I made an incision between two and three inches long in the direction of the tumour, and to my great surprise without any starting, crying, or other indication of pain. The fascia was then divided, the patient still appearing wholly insensible. Then followed the insulation of the veins, during which he began to move his limbs, cry out, and utter extraordinary expressions. These phenomena led to a doubt of the success of the application; and in truth I was not satisfied myself, until I had, soon after the operation and on various other occasions, asked the question whether he had suffered pain. To this he always replied in the negative, adding, however, that he knew of the operation, and comparing the stroke of the knife to that of a blunt instrument passed roughly across his neck.[12]

At the close of the operation Warren is said to have remarked to the spectators, 'Gentlemen, this is no humbug'.

Morton is commonly regarded as the discoverer of inhalation anaesthesia; and, if the credit is to go to one man, it should go to Morton. On the other hand, inhalation anaesthesia was by no means a new idea in 1846, and others had succeeded with it before. Others, too, had realised its enormous possibilities, and had tried to interest fellow doctors and scientists. Where they failed, Morton succeeded. But he owed a great deal to those around him: to Wells, who had given him the idea, save for the use of ether as the agent; to an alert and well-trained chemist named Charles Jackson who gave Morton information and advice about ether which the latter valued; and who subsequently claimed the discovery as his own; to the instrument maker who provided the successful flask inhaler – this was a truly original and important contribution; and not least to Warren, the surgeon at the Massachusetts General Hospital who, having seen Wells fail, was nevertheless prepared to encourage another attempt. If ever a discovery was owed not to one individual working in isolation but to an individual working in a favourable social context, inhalation anaesthesia was that discovery. As Morton himself very honestly said, 'I have got here a little and there a little.' He had and needed the right kind of friends, rivals, associates and nearby institutions; he had around him receptive minds and skilled support; and his achievement was the outcome of all of this. It brought him little happiness. Instead of developing his discovery he tried to patent it, and the world revolted against the idea of the great blessing of ether anaesthesia 'as a secret medicine'. Neglecting his dental practice, he spent years in the attempt to establish his claim to priority and, as a result of this, to the securing of some financial reward. In 1868 he died in poverty. Twenty years previously, Horace Wells, his work overshadowed by the claims and counter-claims of Jackson and Morton, violently disappointed and mentally disturbed, had committed suicide.

A paper describing the 'new anodyne process, by means of which surgical operations have been performed without pain' was read before the Boston Society of Medical Improvement on 9 November 1846, an abstract having been previously read before the American Academy of Arts and Sciences on 3 November. This paper, of about 3,000 words, announced that 'a patient has been rendered completely insensible during an amputation of the thigh, regaining consciousness after a short interval. Other severe operations have been performed without the knowledge of the patients.' The author, Henry Jacob Bigelow, son of the Professor of Materia Medica at Harvard, described four dental operations carried out at Morton's rooms, ether having been administered by means of 'a small two-necked glass globe . . . together with sponges' and a valve in the mouthpiece to divert the expired air. He also raised the question 'whether no accidents have attended the employment of a method so wide in its application, and so striking in its results', and referred to the cases of 'an elderly woman [who] was made to inhale the vapour for at least half an hour without effect', and of a young man whose pulse after 25 minutes' inhalation during a

protracted eye operation, fell from 120 to 96. His respiration became
slow and his hands cold. These symptoms remained unaltered for 15
minutes, and 'active exercise, as in a case of narcotism from opium'
was required to restore consciousness 'at the expiration of an hour'.
Nausea and vomiting were also reported. Bigelow concluded that 'the
process is obviously adapted to operations which are brief in their
duration, whatever be their severity. . . In protracted dissections, the
pain of the first incision alone is of sufficient importance to induce its
use; and it may hereafter prove safe to administer it for a length of time,
and to produce a narcotism of an hour's duration.'

This paper was reprinted, in its entirety, in the *Lancet* of 2 January
1847, having been sent by Professor Bigelow of Harvard to Dr Francis
Boott, an  Englishman educated at Harvard, with a medical degree
from Edinburgh, who was then practising in London. Bigelow's letter
accompanying his son's paper, also printed in the *Lancet*, referred to 'a
new anodyne process lately introduced here, which promises to be one
of the most important discoveries of the present age. It has rendered
many patients insensible to pain during surgical operations, and other
causes of suffering. Limbs and breasts have been amputated, arteries tied,
tumours extirpated, and many hundreds of teeth extracted, without
any consciousness of the least pain on the part of the patient.' Besides
printing this material, the *Lancet* drew particular attention to it by de-
voting one of its two leaders to the subject. Bigelow's paper was 'an
important communication . . . describing the important discovery of
an apparently harmless means of producing insensibility during the performance of surgical operations', and the writer promised (not very
grammatically) to 'watch its development in the various branches of
medicine and surgery which may admit of its application, and carefully
record them'. Recognition of the possible importance of Morton's discovery concluded on a familiar note: 'We suppose we shall now hear no
more of mesmerism and its absurdities as preparatives for surgical
operations. The destruction of one limb of the mesmeric quackery will
be one not inconsiderable merit of this most valuable discovery.' And in
the same issue, a reader still in doubt as to the reality and practicability
of the new discovery could read the following advertisement:

The Inhaler, for Sulphuric Ether Vapour, most perfectly constructed
in accordance with the experience of Dr Boott and Mr Robinson,
will be ready for sale at the beginning of next week, by Mr Hooper,
Operative Chemist, 7, Pall-mall East (opposite the Royal College of
Physicians). Dec 31st, 1846.

It thus must be said that the British response was exceedingly prompt. Bigelow's letter took three weeks to cross the Atlantic, but when at last it came into his hands Boott at once appreciated its significance and lost no time in making use of the information. On 19 December, at Boott's house in Gower Street, a young woman was successfully anaesthetised and a tooth extracted by a Mr Robinson, using ether in an apparatus employing a ball-and-socket valve. (The same apparatus failed 'in three or four cases afterwards'.) Boott wrote at once to Robert Liston, giving him the news, and on 21 December at University College Hospital Liston used ether with success in two operations, amputation of the thigh and evulsion of both sides of the great toe-nail, in both cases using an inhaler 'contrived by Mr Squires, of Oxford Street'.[13] Later the same day, Liston wrote to Boott as follows:

> My Dear Sir;    I tried the ether inhalation today in a case of amputation of the thigh, and in another requiring evulsion of both sides of the great toe-nail, one of the most painful operations in surgery, and with the most perfect and satisfactory results.
>
> It is a very great matter to be able thus to destroy sensibility to such an extent, and without, apparently, any bad result. It is a fine thing for operating surgeons, and I thank you most sincerely for the early information you were so kind as to give me of it.

Among the witnesses of these two operations was Joseph Lister, then a young medical student of nineteen.

The surgeons at University College were as prompt to spread the news as their colleagues in Boston. Within a few weeks operations using ether were reported from as far afield as Maidstone, Bristol, Liverpool and Edinburgh, as well as from every important London hospital. At Guy's the theatre on the first few occasions was 'densely crowded' and at St Bartholomew's 'much crowded by practitioners as well as students'.[14] Only one failure to achieve narcotism was mentioned. Meanwhile, on 16 January, the *Lancet* carried a second and this time lengthy leader on the subject, again emphasising its importance but raising a number of doubts. Ether had hitherto been used as an anti-hysterical remedy, a toy, or a narcotic poison. It might now be possible to use it 'in some cases of operative midwifery; but here it would have to be tried with the utmost care and caution, owing to the tendency to convulsions belonging to the puerperal state'. Secondly, although ether

eliminated pain in operations it did not necessarily follow that it also
eliminated shock; and if operations were to produce shock even in the
absence of pain, 'it will then come to be an important question,
whether an operation performed with great rapidity produces a lesser or
greater shock than one performed with some deliberation. . . It must be
confessed that this question has been in some measure lost sight of,
and that celerity has been the prime and great object with operative
surgeons.' Lastly, there was the question, destined to cause an enormous amount of controversy, whether or not

> the existence [more exactly, the experience] of physical pain may
> excite some physiological action beneficial to the patient. We may
> take an instance of this from parturition. Where there is danger
> of laceration, the pain excites the patient to cry out, and when
> the cry opens the glottis and emits the air of the chest, the thorax
> is no longer a fixed point for the muscular actions, so that a sudden
> removal of the pressure, threatening laceration, occurs. This instance
> is sufficient to show that even pain is not in all cases an unmitigated
> curse.

These points were both sensible and important; but in the following
months they did not receive much in the way of an answer. Simpson
used ether in obstetric cases in Edinburgh from the second half of
January onwards, with success; but although he published on the subject he did not report his cases in the *Lancet,* and probably few medical
men in London knew anything about this aspect of his work. On the
other hand, in March 1847 the *Lancet* published a report from Baron
Dubois, Clinical Professor of Midwifery in Paris, outlining five obstetric cases using ether. There were, he stated, no ascertainable ill-effects
attributable to the ether, either in mother or child. Two of the patients
died, but almost certainly not as a result of anaesthesia. In one case the
patient's face became 'intensely red' and 'the conjunctiva became con-
gested to that degree that I really could imagine blood on the point of
springing from its surface'. But after three minutes the patient recovered. In spite of these not unfavourable experiences, Dubois concluded that to use ether 'frequently' in obstetrics 'would be extremely
imprudent'. Pain and parturition were inseparable. Labour lasted a long
time and to try to anaesthetise a patient for more than a short time
would be 'guilty temerity'. His evidence, as far as it went, was in favour
of ether in operative midwifery, but he was himself, on the whole,
against it. The questions about shock and pain raised in the January

leader remained unanswered, although reports of successful cases of etherisation continued to appear.

Also in March came the report of the death of a young woman at Grantham, allegedly due to the use of ether. The operation had lasted for 55 minutes with the patient lying face downwards. Only the operator himself and an old woman had been present, and no one had been in a position to see the patient's face and observe her breathing. That etherisation was not the cause of death, in spite of the coroner's verdict, was fairly evident, but this fatality (and possibly others like it) may have prompted the *Lancet* to try again to secure more and better information. A leader on 10 April stated that, although 'the number of surgical operations in some of our hospitals has more than doubled' since the introduction of etherisation, many surgeons remain 'profoundly and obdurately silent' on the subject. This silence, it was said, 'has excited much astonishment throughout the profession'. The writer did not ask why, in spite of the accumulation of experience from 'many hundreds of cases', so little discussion took place. Was it because surgeons grasped at the possibility of eliminating pain and wished to close their eyes to the possible harmful or even disastrous consequences? Or was it because they had no idea of what the possible consequences might be? Or was it because several fatal cases involving the use of ether had already taken place, and the profession was not anxious to publicise or discuss them? No answer can be given to these questions, which may or may not have been behind the *Lancet's* thirst for more information. But to ask for the facts – 'full and ample particulars' – was the right course, and notice was given that Mr Wakley, junior surgeon to the Royal Free Hospital and eldest son of the reforming and controversial founder and editor of the *Lancet,* was to set up an enquiry. Wakley proposed to circulate surgeons in all the metropolitan and country hospitals, asking for 'strictly accurate evidence' about etherisation. His questionnaire, reproduced in the journal, includes questions about the nature and duration of the operation, the age of the patient, the temperature of body and room, the nature of the apparatus, the diameter of the air passages, the kind of ether used, the nature of the effects, the state of the pulse, and so on. It is or should have been a useful document although it makes no reference curiously to the dose or duration of inhalation. Unfortunately, no account exists of the response to this questionnaire, if indeed it was ever issued.

The British debate on etherisation, such as it was, was overtaken by events. Immediately after the first successful British operation, Liston wrote to an old colleague, James Miller, Professor of Surgery at Edinburgh, telling him that with the use of ether 'a new light had burst on surgery, and a large boon [been] conferred on mankind'. Miller read the letter to his surgical class on 23 December, having the previous day, in all probability, given the news to his next-door neighbour. This neighbour was James Young Simpson, and this was his first knowledge of inhalation anaesthesia.

In 1846 Simpson was 35 years of age, Professor of Midwifery at Edinburgh. He had been born at Bathgate, then a small market town 15 miles west of Edinburgh, where his parents had run the local bakery. He was the seventh child in a family very far from rich, although not as poor as most, and as a boy he helped his mother and father by riding round the cottages to deliver the early morning rolls and bread. That he was bright and intelligent was early obvious, and, as was common in Scotland in those days, the family was prepared to make sacrifices to send one child to the university. In 1825, at the age of 14, Simpson arrived in Edinburgh, feeling 'very very young and very solitary, very poor and almost friendless', and enrolled in the classes of Junior Greek and Humanity. He digged — that is to say, lodged — in the top floor of an old tenement in Stockbridge with a slightly senior school-fellow from Bathgate who was a medical student. The two boys rose early, worked late, and lived exceedingly simply. In 1827 Simpson abandoned his classical studies, which would probably have led him into the Church, and took up medicine.

Medical education in Scotland in the first half of the nineteenth century was much better organised and more effective than in England. The famous Edinburgh medical school had come into existence in the 1720s, founded by a small group of professors who had studied at what was then the most advanced centre of medical learning in Europe, the University of Leyden. The Edinburgh system depended on courses of lectures which were well planned and co-ordinated, given by the professors, and covering some basic science as well as the essential medical subjects such as anatomy, materia medica, and physics. There was also organised clinical teaching, and a lengthy final examination at the end of three years. This was the system which, along with the services of a number of unusually able men, made Edinburgh and Glasgow in the later decades of the eighteenth century 'undoubtedly the greatest medical schools in Britain, and probably in Europe'.[15] Edinburgh, in particular, enjoyed an international reputation. In the 1830s and 1840s approximately half its medical graduates were from Scotland, one-third from England, and the remainder from 'the colonies'.

When Simpson began his medical studies in 1827, however, the situation was not quite as favourable as it had been in the eighteenth century. One visitor in 1803 even 'turned a look of pity towards Edinburgh, and sighed over the fallen condition and lamented the decaying state of the medical school'.[16] This was hardly reasonable behaviour, however, or fair comment; and one of his criticisms, that Edinburgh was 'degrading [medicine] to a mechanical and a dirty trade' must seem today to be a compliment, reflecting Edinburgh's recognition of the connection between medicine and the methods of experimental science. But there were difficulties. The supply of corpses for dissection was inadequate – the efforts of Burke and Hare in the 1820s were directed towards meeting a real need. Part of the examination at Edinburgh consisted of a thesis, and there is evidence that the grinders – those who supplied tuition outside the walls and outside the control of the university – not only provided medical students with information and answers to possible questions, but also corrected theses which would not have satisfied the examiners, or, in the extreme case, wrote the students' theses themselves. Examinations and theses were in Latin – a change to English, it was held, would 'open a door for the graduation . . . of illiterate and impudent empyricks'[17] – and this may have favoured those who were better at languages than at medicine. What is worse, it seems doubtful whether the best men were now being appointed to Chairs. 'Between 1786 and 1807 ten appointments to Medical Chairs were made and in eight of these the son of an Edinburgh medical professor was appointed.'[18] The most celebrated case is that of Monro Tertius, Professor of Anatomy from 1808 to 1846. His father and grandfather had held the Chair before him, with distinction. But Monro Tertius was a nonentity who, said Charles Darwin, 'made his lectures on human anatomy as dull as he was himself, and the subject disgusted me'.[19] Moreover, several of these nineteenth-century professors seem to have been less interested in lecturing to the students than their eighteenth-century predecessors had been, and more interested in private practice; one of the most celebrated of them, James Gregory, Professor of the Institutes of Medicine, explained to the Senate in 1819 that attending to his patients sometimes meant that his lectures were 'interrupted for several days, nay even for weeks together'.[20] It was probably this sort of behaviour that led to the extensive development of extra-mural teaching in the basic subjects, especially anatomy. Much of this extra-mural teaching was of a high standard; but its practitioners did not, any more than the professor, do the kind of work that would advance the frontiers of medical knowledge, and make students feel that they were in contact with the search for new ideas.

Nevertheless, the education provided was by the standards of the day a very good one, and an enthusiastic and enterprising student was in a position to acquire a good knowledge of contemporary medicine and surgery. Simpson became a licentiate of the Royal College of Surgeons, Edinburgh, in 1829, but being only 18 years old he was too young to take his MD. He had already, in vacations, assisted the country doctor in Bathgate, and now he took a job assisting a Dr Gardiner in Edinburgh, and at the same time attended a course of extra-mural lectures in midwifery, a subject not then compulsory for graduation. In 1832 he presented himself for the MD examination. He was required to answer questions on medicine and surgery (all in Latin), to comment on two aphorisms of Hippocrates, and to defend his thesis, which was entitled *De Causa Mortis in Quileusdam Inflammationibus Proxima*. This was the normal form of the MD examination. The examiners were satisfied, and one of them, the Professor of Pathology, was so well satisfied that he forthwith engaged Simpson as his assistant; and thus, as Simpson himself later wrote, 'I came to settle down a citizen of Edinburgh and fight amongst you the hard and uphill battle of life for bread and name and fame. . .'[21]

Simpson had a hard and uphill battle in as far as he came, so to speak, from nowhere. He was a country loon without connections or influence of any kind, and he had to make his own way in the world. On the other hand, his warm and lively personality, in addition to his obvious intelligence, quickly gained him friends of all ages, and in all walks of life. He was an engaging fellow. As a boy of 14 he caught the eye of the Professor of Humanity, who encouraged him to compete for a small bursary which Simpson won. As a doctor's assistant in Bathgate he was remembered as 'a pleasant tempered, laughingly inclined lad'.[22] The assistantship he obtained in 1832 must have depended on the personal impression he made upon the Professor of Pathology, at least as much as on his thesis itself. It was said of him in later life that he had 'no acquaintances, only friends'; and although he also had enemies, the general truth of the observation is undeniable.

The Professor of Pathology who gave Simpson his first job also gave him a piece of advice: 'It was at Dr Thompson's urgent suggestion and advice that I first turned my attention more especially to the study of Midwifery, with a view to becoming a teacher in this department'. Midwifery was held in low esteem in the early decades of the nineteenth century, and in Scotland there was still widespread dislike of 'men-midwives'. But by the 1830s the medical profession was just beginning to take obstetrics seriously, and Simpson's decision, from a career point of view, was a wise one. Having determined that this was to be his future, Simpson attended a course of lectures by James Hamilton, the Professor of Midwifery, and with this Professor (who used to go about in one of the last sedan chairs to be seen in the streets of Edinburgh) he also became friendly. His own lectures on pathology continued and were going well. And in 1835, having borrowed the required money from one of his brothers, he went off on a continental tour. He spent 'a most happy and instructive month' in London visiting numerous hospitals as well as a meeting of the Linnaeian Society. In France he met many French doctors and surgeons, and heard them discuss their cases. He was greatly taken by France, entranced by the strange customs of the people and by the still more unusual clothes of the fishermen, the customs officers, and postilions and, above all, the women. Returning to Edinburgh in the summer of 1835 he was elected President of the Royal Medical Society — a coveted honour for a rising young doctor — and gave his inaugural dissertation on *The Diseases of the Placenta*.

This paper is an important indication of Simpson's methods of thought, and indeed of his attitude to medicine. In preparing it he wrote to many physicians whom he had met in France, and to many others whom he had never met, in England, Belgium and Germany. He dug out information from obscure and venerable volumes, and accumulated references to works by British, Irish, French, German, Italian and American authors. He surveyed an enormous amount of evidence (some of it of a most doubtful character) digested it, arranged it, and commented on it. What he wrote was in no way experimental, and in a sense it was scarcely even original. His principal conclusion was that, in cases of placental congestion and inflammation, 'general blood-letting, repeated or not, according to circumstances, along with more or fewer other antiphlogistic measures, has been long successfully employed . . . and [this enquiry shows] the value and rational character of this practice . . . also it would seem not unreasonable to anticipate that . . . an active employment of leeching . . . may be attended with highly beneficial results'. The paper, published in the *Edinburgh Medical and Surgical Journal* in April 1836, was a great success. It was translated into French, German and Italian, and at the age of 25 Simpson became an acknowledged authority on what was grudgingly admitted to be an important subject.

After the publication of this paper Simpson decided to lecture on midwifery — 'I believe teaching the subject to others the best way to teach oneself' — and he again borrowed from his family, this time in order to set up as an extra-mural lecturer. Also — and this too was after the publication of his paper, not before — he began to practise midwifery. He took a part-time position at the Lying-in Hospital, moved to a more fashionable address, and began to build up a practice. He also continued to publish, contributing to the medical journals of the day, in London as well as in Edinburgh, many more papers than was then usual for a member of the medical faculty. By the end of the 1830s he was established as the principal teacher and practitioner of midwifery in Edinburgh, with a large practice that kept him busy principally in the poorer but also increasingly in the wealthier districts of the town. When Hamilton resigned his Chair in 1839, Simpson was the obvious successor.

The Edinburgh Chair of Midwifery was the oldest in the British Isles, having been established in 1726. The Medical Faculty at that time had not wanted it, and arguments about whether or not it should be retained, and if it were retained who should have the right to appoint to it, were recurrent. In the 1820s a dispute arose between the Medical Faculty and the Town Council as to whether or not midwifery was essential for graduation in medicine. The Town Council held that it was, the Medical Faculty that it was not. Unenthusiastic about the subject, the medical professors nevertheless held strong views about who should occupy the Chair, and in 1839, the Town Council having established its right to make the appointment, they left no stone unturned in their efforts to influence the Council's decision. They were decidedly averse to Simpson's appointment. He was too young; he was not married; and — although this was not said in so many words — he was ambitious, bustling, unconventional, and not always respectful to his seniors. Moreover, he was disliked by James Syme, Professor of Clinical Surgery and the most distinguished member of the Medical School. Undaunted, Simpson launched a campaign to defeat the efforts of his rivals and to win over the Town Council. He wrote letters to all and sundry soliciting support and he drew up a lengthy *curriculum vitae* which he had printed and posted to all those who he thought might be able to influence the Town Councillors. This document included a list of his publications along with favourable comments on his work by students and authorities in the field of midwifery, both at home and overseas. In order to put an end to the objection that it was indelicate if not improper for an unmarried man to be an obstetrician, he married. And in order to finance all these proceedings, he borrowed money, this time from his father-in-law. These efforts were successful, and at the beginning of 1840 Simpson was elected to the Chair by a majority of one.

Thus, within less than eight years of graduation, Simpson – 'a poor baker's son', as he once described himself – become a professor in a distinguished school of medicine. What may well have been a youthful dream was already realised. He was 28 – not the youngest man ever appointed to a medical chair at Edinburgh, but one of the youngest. He had worked hard, he was popular among the townspeople both rich and poor, he had a considerable reputation, even on the continent; but he had not yet contributed anything very remarkable to medicine. A lesser man, striving merely for title and place, might have been content. But Simpson was not a lesser man. He had a sense of mission, and an endlessly enquiring mind. He was restless, energetic, tireless and companionable. If he entered a dull or awkward company, it was said, 'in a few minutes, under the genial influence of his presence, all tongues are set a-wagging'. He liked people, and he believed in work. In 1842 he gave the newly qualified medical students at Edinburgh this advice:

> In entering upon the active duties of Medical Practitioners, form your earlier habits of business and study with anxious and watchful care . . . Above all, teach yourselves carefully to save your time, and to methodize all your pursuits. . . Look around the profession, and you will find that those who have most to do in the way of business as practitioners, have also apparently the most time to spare as observers and writers, in contributing to the literature and advancing the knowledge both of our science and art. . . Do everything in its proper season, and you will have time to do everything slowly and well. Have a duty for every time, and you will have time for every duty.[23]

> Do not wait for special and favourable circumstances, but work always as if special and favourable circumstances were already actually present. Do not withold your blows till the iron is heated, but 'strike it till it becomes hot'. Never spare yourselves in your efforts.[24]

This was the ethic of work; Victorian, or Presbyterian, or both. And what one worked for was not just money:

> Your aim is, as far as possible, to alleviate human suffering, and

lengthen out human existence. Your ambition is to gladden as well as prolong the course of human life . . . [but] if you practice the art that you profess with a cold-hearted view to its results merely as a matter of lucre and trade, your course will be as dark and miserable as that low and grovelling lust that dictates it.[25]

Simpson made money, but he never sought it. Long after he was established as one of the most popular doctors in Edinburgh with patients in every part of the town — by the 1840s his private practice alone was more than enough work for one ordinary individual — he was still, as his wife remarked, 'apt to spend his time with the poor and forget to collect the fees due to him from his richer patients'. He was not interested in money, but he cared for people, and in a typically Scots fashion he cared for them without distinction of rank or class. In his practice, said the professor of Obstetrics at Harvard who visited Simpson in 1852,

> are the poor and the rich together, with no other distinctions than such as will best accommodate both. And I can say, from a long and wide observation, that there is no difference in their treatment.[26]

At the heart of Simpson's conduct lay a great and simple kindliness; he was, in the fullest sense of the word, a most charitable man. It was the custom in those days for the doctor to receive his fee when the consultation ended, 'and by offering the hand for farewell, the fee is deposited in his'. But Simpson did not always accept it. 'I have seen him press the guinea, for that it usually is, back into the hand of the patient with a "na, na, awa' with ye".'[27]

A multitude of human contacts in a rapidly growing practice did not diminish Simpson's intellectual activity. He had a boundless curiosity. He wrote on the incidence of leprosy in Great Britain, starting well before the Middle Ages; on the importance of pathology in medicine; on homeopathy; on the rate of mortality after amputations in hospitals; on syphilis in Scotland in the fifteenth and sixteenth centuries; on the alleged infecundity of females born co-twins with males; as well as on a large variety of obstetrical and gynaecological subjects. Partly as a consequence of his writing, but probably more because of his sympathetic and innovative management of women in labour, Simpson's influence on the practice of midwifery began to be considerable. It was a field of medicine that badly needed some new ideas.

In Burns's *Textbook of Midwifery,* the most enlightened handbook of the period, blood-letting, purgation and opiates were the standard remedies to obstetrical problems and lubrication with lard a ready answer to the tedious labour. No wonder Simpson's waiting room was rather crowded with women desperate to consult someone whom they had heard was prepared to try something else.[28]

He invented − or reinvented − the uterine sound, and was the first to use it diagnostically for parts usually considered beyond the reach of examination. Shortly after this he devised a complicated method, long since superseded, to achieve 'dilation of the uteric cavity for a variety of purposes and indications'. These advances arose from Simpson's interest not solely in problems of childbirth but also in wider gynaecological problems, in the extreme case in questions of operative gynaecology. In these fields Simpson was making, along with some continental colleagues, a significant extension to the scope of medical enquiry and practice.

Both his work and his publications brought him into frequent conflict with his fellow professors. There was nothing unusual in this. When Simpson's predecessor James Hamilton published an attack on his colleagues in 1927 ('His language was apt to be unmeasured, whence quarrels arose'[29]) Professor James Gregory − whose 'most abiding monument in the temple of fame is a powder containing rhubarb, magnesia and ginger, which has been perhaps more universally employed than any other pharmacopoeial preparation'[30] − assaulted the vituperative Hamilton with his walking-stick, and subsequently had to pay £100 damages. When Liston quite reasonably criticised the manager of the Royal Infirmary in 1822 they responded by 'prohibiting Mr Liston from entering the wards or operation room of the Royal Infirmary at any time, on any pretence whatever'.[31] Liston was at this time probably already the most distinguished surgeon in Britain. After his death in 1848 his place was to be taken by James Syme who in the 1820s was a very young surgeon, a man of obvious promise and enormous independence of mind. Liston and Syme were in Edinburgh together and were at first on good terms; but they 'became less cordial' in the later 1820s, and their differences 'proceeded to such a height, and they raised so much acrimony between their opposing factions, that when Syme applied for the surgeonship of the Royal Infirmary the managers declined to appoint him lest he and Liston should quarrel openly in the institution, and their rival students disturb its peace'.[32] As his colleagues behaved, so did Simpson; he never shrank from a fight, and he made no false pretences to politeness. In 1839, for example, he admitted to the Lock Hospital a most wretched young woman who had contracted venereal disease for the second time. This admission was against the rules, and the Reverend Lachlan McLean, the Superior, protested. One of Simpson's letters to this gentleman is as follows:

Dear Sir,
The nature of your profession prevents me from answering your letter in the mode which it deserves.

Your obedient servant,

James Y. Simpson, MD

On another occasion, in the midst of some differences with Syme, Simpson met the great surgeon when both men were called to the same case by the family doctor. Accused of meddling in matters he did not understand, Simpson was not at a loss for a reply, and for a short time the most distinguished surgeon and the most distinguished obstetrician in Britain stood exchanging insults on the patient's doorstep. As an eminent surgeon of the following generation was wont to remark, 'they were giants in those days; but they were very quarrelsome giants'.[33]

Such was the Professor of Midwifery who learnt at the end of 1846 that inhalation anaesthesia was a practical proposition. 'It is a glorious thought', he wrote, 'I can think of naught else'. He was, as his most recent biographer remarks, 'always on to something new',[34] and he at once went to London and saw Liston, who presumably confirmed that ether could be used successfully in surgery. But what Simpson wanted to know was, could it be used successfully in child-birth? A surgical operation lasted for minutes, but labour might last for hours. Prolonged anaesthesia might prove injurious or fatal; Liston himself believed that the principal use of chloroform anaesthesia would be in operations lasting only a few minutes. Moreover, it was possible that administering ether might cause the uterine contractions to weaken or stop, or might result in some unanticipated damage to mother or child. As no one understood the physiology of anaesthetic action, only two courses were open; to wait for more scientific knowledge, or to risk it. Simpson risked it. He had a patient, 'lame and deformed' with a contracted pelvis whose labour pains began on 19 January 1847. Her first labour had continued 'upwards of three days', and finally, in an operation lasting for more than an hour, the child had been drawn out in pieces. On this occasion, Simpson administered ether before turning the child.

> During the whole operation, she was (according to her own sub-
> sequent reiterated declaration and surprise) quite unaware of feeling
> any pain, or having any sensation whatever, and awoke just as the
> delivery was being terminated. One of her first recollections was
> regarding the bustle of preparing a bath for the child. After she was
> brought under the influence of the ether, the uterine contractions
> continued regularly, but without knowledge or consciousness of pain
> on the patient's part. She is making the best possible recovery.[35]

This was possibly but not certainly the first time that inhalation anaesthesia was used in childbirth. The Professor of Obstetrics at Harvard
already referred to, Dr Channing, stated in 1848 that he had used anaesthetics 'for many years', but the meaning of this statement is not clear.

As 1847 wore on, Simpson used ether with increasing confidence
and increasing frequency:

> Since the latter part of January I have employed etherization, with
> few and rare exceptions, in every case of labour which has been
> under my care. And the results . . . have been, indeed, most happy
> and gratifying. I never had the pleasure of watching over a series of
> more perfect or more rapid recoveries; nor have I witnessed any dis-
> agreeble result to either mother or child.[36]

Yet there were difficulties. Ether was apt to irritate the eyes, had an
objectionable smell and sometimes caused vomiting. The amount of
liquid needed to bring about loss of consciousness was not great, but
it was another matter when prolonged anaesthesia was required, as in
childbirth; and this was a serious practical inconvenience in a society
in which many children were born at home; carrying a large heavy
glass bottle up dirty, stone, tenement stairs to the sixth or seventh
floor — not uncommon in Edinburgh — would have made any obstetrician ask himself if some other agent could not be found. Moreover,
ether was inflammable; it could be dangerous if held too near a light;
and in the 1840s houses were lit either by gaslight or by candlelight,
and there were coal fires in the rooms. Most serious of all, there was
no certainty that the use of ether was absolutely safe in childbirth.
Even in 1847 cases began to be reported involving the use of ether,
and in which the mother had died; and no one could be sure that
in these cases ether was not at least a contributory cause of death. A

French physician, himself a pioneer in the use of ether in childbirth, wrote in 1847:

> My profound feeling on the subject is, that inhalation of ether in midwifery should be restrained to a very limited number of cases, the nature of which . . . experience will better allow us to determine.[37]

Simpson must have known of and indeed have shared some of these doubts and objections, because, although he continued to use ether and to advocate its use by others, he began at an early date to look out for some alternative anaesthetic.

During 1847 many doctors were at work trying to obtain a better and a safer agent than ether. Thomas Nunneley experimented systematically with over 40 substances and discovered several new anaesthetics, but they were either dangerous, or expensive and difficult to produce. Half-way through the year Sir William Lawrence at St Bartholomew's was using an agent known to him as chloric ether, i.e. chloroform dissolved in rectified spirit; had he had the requisite knowledge of chemistry, he could have concentrated this chloric ether and obtained chloroform. John Snow, a brilliant experimental scientist and physician, was also working on the problem. In this company Simpson had few advantages except boldness and energy. He knew as much physiology as the next man (which was not much in 1847) but rather little chemistry; and he was certainly not, by training or inclination, an experimental scientist. One of his comments on ether was, 'I have taken it myself to try its effects. It is the only way of judging it', and this was the path along which he proceeded. He tried inhaling a whole series of volatile fluids — acetone, ethyl nitrate, benzin, vapour of iodform, and so on. The process was anything but safe, as one of his suppliers, the Professor of Chemistry at Edinburgh, later testified:

> On one occasion he came into my laboratory to ask whether I had any new substance likely to produce anaesthesia. My assistant, Dr Guthrie, had just prepared a volatile liquid, bibromide of ethylene, which I thought worthy of experiment. Simpson, who was brave to rashness in his experiments, wished to try it upon himself in my private room. This I absolutely refused to allow, and declined to give him any of the liquid unless he promised me first to try its effects on rabbits. Two were procured, and under the vapour quickly passed into anaesthesia, coming out of it in due

course. Next day Simpson proposed to experiment upon himself and his assistant with this liquid, but the latter suggested that
they should first see how the rabbits had fared. They were both
found to be dead...[38]

In October Simpson was visited by an acquaintance of his student days,
David Waldie, who suggested that it might be worth trying pure chloroform. Chloroform had been discovered in an impure state in 1831 by
Soubeiran in France and simultaneously by Samuel Guthrie working in
America. Guthrie, however, failed to realise that the properties of
chloroform were not the same as those of the already known chloride
of hydro-carbon, and neither he nor Soubeiran investigated its possibilities as an anaesthetic. In 1834 it was correctly analysed by Dumas in
France, and named. It was occasionally used in medicine, and was prescribed at one time or another in the 1830s and 1840s for asthma,
hysteria, cancer and neuralgia. In 1842 a young Edinburgh graduate
showed that it was a powerful narcotic poison to animals and could
produce insensibility, and this was further demonstrated by the French
physiologist, P.J.H. Flourens in 1847. Simpson probably knew rather
little of all this, but Waldie, who was a professional chemist, may have
known a good deal; some years later it was even suggested by an extremely well-informed contemporary that 'when [Dr Waldie] informed
Dr Simpson of the existence and nature of chloroform, he was able to
give him, not merely an opinion, but an almost certain knowledge of
its effects'.[39] This may be true. But the fact remains that almost certain
knowledge is not conclusive proof, and that although he owed something to others just as Morton had done, Simpson was justified in his
subsequent statement that 'on the 15th November, 1847, the anaesthetic effects of chloroform were discovered [i.e. finally established in
surgery] in Edinburgh'.

The account of the initial discovery given by Professor Miller, Simpson's next-door neighbour, has often been quoted, but it bears repetition as a crystal-clear flashback to one of the most astonishing, and
'unscientific', moments in the history of medicine:

Late one evening — it was the 4th of November, 1847 — on returning home after a weary day's labour, Dr Simpson, with his two
friends and assistants, Drs Keith and Matthew Duncan, sat down to
their somewhat hazardous work in Dr Simpson's dining room.
Having inhaled several substances, but without much effect, it
occurred to Dr Simpson to try a ponderous material, which he had

formerly set aside on a lumber table, and which, on account of its great weight, he had hitherto regarded as of no likelihood whatever. That happened to be a small bottle of chloroform. It was searched for, and recovered from beneath a heap of waste paper. And with each tumbler newly charged, the inhalers resumed their vocation. Immediately an unwonted hilarity seized the party; they become bright-eyed, very happy and very loquacious — expatiating on the delicious aroma of the new fluid. The coversation was of unusual intelligence, and quite charmed the listeners — some ladies of the family and a naval officer, brother-in-law of Dr Simpson. But suddenly there was talk of sounds being heard like those of a cotton mill, louder and louder; a moment more, then all was quiet, and then — a crash. On awaking, Dr Simpson's first perception was mental — 'This is far stronger and better than ether', said he to himself. His second was to note that he was prostrate on the floor, and that among the friends about him there was both confusion and alarm. Hearing a noise, he turned round and saw Dr Duncan beneath a chair. . . snoring in a most determined and alarming manner. . . And then his eyes overtook Dr Keith's feet and legs, making valorous efforts to overturn the supper table, or more probably to annihilate everything that was on it. . .[40]

Whatever others had done or suggested previously, this was certainly the first time that chloroform was successfully used on human beings deliberately to produce insensibility.

Characteristically, Simpson lost no time in putting his discovery to use. He forthwith 'exhibited it with perfect success in tooth-drawing, opening abscesses, for annulling the pain of dysmenorrhoea and of neuralgia . . . etc'.[41] On 8 November he first used chloroform in an obstetrical case (half a teaspoon of liquid was poured into a pocket handkerchief rolled into a funnel shape) and again with complete success:

The child was born in about twenty-five minutes after the inhalation had begun. The mother subsequently remained longer, I think, stuperose than commonly happens after ether. The squalling of the child did not arouse her; and some minutes elapsed after the placenta was expelled, and after the child was removed by the nurse into another room, before the patient awoke.[42]

A week later Simpson administered chloroform to three surgical cases in the Royal Infirmary, and again the results were completely satisfactory. (On the previous day Miller had been ready to try chloroform in a case of strangulated hernia, but Simpson was not available to administer it. The operation proceeded, and the patient died before it was completed. Had chloroform been administered in this case, and had the result been the same, acceptance of chloroform as an anaesthetic would almost certainly have been seriously delayed.)

Before these operations took place, Simpson had already published a pamphlet[43] describing what he called the 'superior anaesthetic properties of chloroform', having, as he said, 'now tried it upon upwards of thirty individuals'. Chloroform was said to possess four advantages over sulphuric ether:

1. A greatly less quantity of Chloroform . . . is requisite to produce the anaesthetic effect. . .
2. Its action is much more rapid and complete, and generally more persistent. . .
3. Most of those who know . . . the sensations produced by ether inhalation, and who have subsequently breathed the Chloroform, have strongly declared the inhalation and influence of Chloroform to be far more agreeable and pleasant than those of Ether. . .
4. I believe that, considering the small quantity requisite, as compared with Ether, the use of Chloroform will be less expensive. . .

Simpson added that no special kind of inhaler or instrument was required. 'A little of the liquid diffused upon the interior of a hollow-shaped sponge, or a pocket-handkerchief, or a piece of linen or paper, and held over the mouth and nostrils, so as to be fully inhaled, generally suffices in about a minute or two to produce the desired effect. After the successful use in surgery on 10 November, Simpson added a postscript on this development also. The pamphlet was published on 15 November and 1,500 copies were sold in less than two weeks. Simpson dedicated it to Professor Dumas, who had given chloroform its name and who, extraordinarily enough, was present at the operations in Edinburgh on the 15th. It bore also the words of Bacon, 'I esteem it the office of a physician not only to restore health, but to mitigate pain and dolor'.

## Notes

1. Thomas Percival (1740–1804), physician. One of the founders of the Manchester Literary and Philosophical Society.

2. J. Priestley, *Directions for Impregnating Water with Fixed Air* (London, 1772), pp. 18–21.

3. Quoted in M. Duncum, *Development of Inhalation Anaesthesia* (Oxford, 1947), pp. 63–4.

4. A generic term for concretions occurring within the body.

5. H. Davy, *Researches, Chemical and Philosophical, Chiefly Concerning Nitrous Oxide* (London, 1800), pp. 458, 460.

6. Ibid., pp. 464–5.

7. Ibid., p. 556.

8. This is suggested in Duncum , *Inhalation Anaesthesia*, pp. 72–3.

9. Quoted in Duncum, *Inhalation Anaesthesia*, p. 77.

10. *Edinburgh University Journal and Critical Review*, No. 11 (January 1823), p. 6.

11. Quoted in Duncum, *Inhalation Anaesthesia*, p. 90.

12. Quoted in Duncum, *Inhalation Anaesthesia*, p. 110.

13. A sponge saturated with ether was contained in a vessel fitted with a flexible tube, leading to a mouthpiece and with a valve to prevent expiration through the vessel. Curiously enough the vessel itself had been originally described and illustrated by Joseph Priestley, but with a quite different purpose in mind.

14. *Lancet*, vol. 1, (1847), p. 105.

15. C. Newman, *The Evolution of Medical Education in the Nineteenth-Century* (Oxford, 1957), p. 13.

16. John Bristed, *Pedestrian Tour*, quoted in D.B. Horn, *A. Short History of the University of Edinburgh* (Edinburgh, 1967), p. 106.

17. Ibid., p. 107.

18. Ibid., p. 108.

19. T.H. Huxley, 'Charles Darwin', in G. de Beer, (ed.) *Autobiographies* (Oxford, 1974), p. 25. The reign of father, son and grandson in the Department of Anatomy lasted, all told, 126 years.

20. Horn, *A Short History of the University of Edinburgh*, p. 107.

21. Quoted in Simpson, *Simpson the Obstetrician*, p. 48.

22. Ibid., p. 46.

23. M. Simpson, *Remarks on the Conduct and Duties of Young Physicians* (Edinburgh, 1842), pp. 6–9.

24. Ibid., p. 12.

25. Ibid., pp. 17–18.

26. W. Channing, *A Physician's Vacation* (Boston, 1856), p. 533.

27. Ibid., p. 190.

28. Simpson, *Simpson the Obstetrician*, p. 100.

29. A. Grant, *Story of the University of Edinburgh*, vol. II (London, 1884), p. 417.

30. J.D. Comrie, *History of Scottish Medicine*, vol. II (London, 1932), p. 475.

31. Comrie, ibid., p. 591.

32. Ibid., p. 593.

33. Sir William Gairdner, quoted in Comrie, *History of Scottish Medicine*, vol. II, p. 645.

34. Simpson, *Simpson the Obstetrician*, p. 120.

35. J.Y. Simpson in *Monthly Journal of Medical Science* (February, 1847), pp. 639–40.

36. J.Y. Simpson, *Remarks of the Superinduction of Anaesthesia in Natural*

*and Morbid Parturition* (Edinburgh, 1847), p. 12.

37. Baron P. Dubois in the *Lancet*, vol. I, (1847), pp. 246–9.

38. Wemyss Reid, *Memoirs and Correspondence of Lord Playfair* (London, 1899), p. 183.

39. J. Snow, *On Chloroform and Other Anaesthetics* (London, 1858), p. 17.

40. James Miller, *The Principles of Surgery* (Philadelphia, 1852), p. 701.

41. J.Y. Simpson, *Account of a New Anaesthetic Agent as a Substitute for Sulphuric Ether in Surgery and Midwifery* (Edinburgh, 1847), p. 5.

42. Ibid.

43. Ibid.

# 3 THE FIGHT FOR CHLOROFORM

Simpson's discovery of chloroform as an anaesthetic gave the world a choice: pain could be alleviated·through the use of chloroform; or it could be alleviated through the use of ether; or it could simply continue without alleviation: and this choice had to be made in respect both of surgery and of midwifery.

At first, it looked as if chloroform would carry all before it. Simpson was convinced that in chloroform he had found an anaesthetic agent 'more portable, more manageable and powerful, more agreeable to inhale, and less exciting' than ether, and one giving 'greater control and command over the superinduction of the anaesthetic state'; and his conviction soon spread. 'The introduction of chloroform', wrote Dr Warren in Boston, 'produced an excitement scarcely less than that of the discovery of the narcotic effect of ether'.[1] In many circles, even in many medical circles, chloroform was within a few months spoken of as if ether had never existed, and Simpson was hailed, principally but not exclusively in Scotland, as the discoverer not only of chloroform anaesthesia, but of anaesthesia itself. All over Europe and in America surgeons began to use chloroform as well as or often instead of ether. This was partly because of its convenience – a small bottle of chloroform would do the work of a large bottle of ether – and partly because the impression arose that chloroform was safer than ether. Simpson had not made this claim; but the confident tone of his pamphlet gave the impression that chloroform was in every way the superior drug.

Some debate as to the relative merits of chloroform and ether did take place. In particular, T.H. Wakley, who had devised the etherisation questionnaire in 1847, called attention to the problem.[2] The relative merit question, he declared, was one 'now claiming from the scientific world . . . an intense degree of attention'. Ether had been adopted 'with almost electrical rapidity', thus proving 'that the medical practitioners of England [sic] and France are worthy of the science they cultivate'. Their actions showed their correct appreciation of ether as 'a blessing conferred on humanity', but its use, he went on,

> . . . is at present of too empirical a character to be satisfactory to a profession where members sincerely and anxiously desire that the *practice* of the science of medicine should be always regulated and

controlled by the *principles* which distinguish that science . . . which of the two is the best agent? Are they both equally safe? Can both be employed on all occasions? These are questions which ought to be, and must be satisfactorily answered. Facts alone can supply the materials which will warrant conclusive replies.

And without further ado this scientific surgeon set some facts on paper. He had carried out, he explained, one hundred experiments on dogs, rats, rabbits, birds, guinea pigs and other creatures, including one she-ass and two mares, using in some cases ether and in other cases chloroform. Of those creatures anaesthetised with ether 21 recovered and 11 died; of those anaesthetised with chloroform 37 recovered and 30 died. The total is 99; Wakley's list does not include experiment no. 58.

What is so remarkable about this performance is, from beginning to end, its hopelessly unscientific character. Besides the she-ass and the two mares and the birds, nine different kinds of animals were subjected to chloroform, but only four kinds to ether; the numbers used varied from two pigs, two guinea pigs and two hedgehogs (all chloroformed) to 33 rats; in no case was the same number of animals anaesthetised with chloroform as with ether (the largest variation was dogs, chloroformed, seventeen; dogs, etherised, one); the animals of the same species varied markedly in size (dogs from ten pounds to forty pounds) and presumably in age and physical condition (one was 'a weakly puppy'); and the dosage varied even for similar animals. Dissections were carried out after death (it is not clearly stated that this was done in all cases) and these showed that 'blood, almost black, had collected in the heart and lungs, and the great vessels connected with these organs' to an astonishing degree. This was held to prove 'obviously and necessarily' that neither chloroform nor ether should be used in a case involving 'any disease of the heart, any aneurism near to the heart, any threatening dyspnoea, or any tendency to an engorgement of the lungs'. Even more surprising, Wakley inferred that, 'in any of the abnormal conditions here described . . . the more dangerous one of the two [agents] would be found in the vapour of chloroform'. For this conclusion the ninety-nine experiments provided no evidence whatever, and Wakley apparently relied (although he did not say so) on another 'fact', namely, that a 'celebrated surgeon' had recently taken chloroform to relieve 'a paroxysm of dyspnoea' and had died, a post-mortem showing that the lungs were 'engorged throughout'.

This contribution might seem so bad as to be not worth mentioning; but it was the only attempt at experimental comparison and was referred to several times by later writers. The general view was that chloroform was on the whole to be preferred to ether, but that Wakley's argument against using chloroform if heart disease was present was a powerful one; and this was believed by many doctors in spite of the fact that congestion of the heart and the lungs after death cannot be a proof of congestion during inhalation, confined within reasonable bounds. Indeed, as one writer pointed out, the arteries are nearly always found empty after death, but this is not taken as proof that they are empty during life. The fact that ether was safer than chloroform was for some years not understood, or not admitted. Ether cannot cause sudden death by paralysis of the heart; a fatality is almost impossible if ether is administered with intelligence and attention. Nevertheless, patients did die under ether, and besides, ether had disadvantages of its own. Many patients found it disagreeable to inhale, and vomiting after recovery was common − more common although less prolonged than after chloroform. Moreover, many doctors believed that etherisation increased the tendency to haemorrhage. To induce insensibility, eight or ten times as much ether might be required as chloroform, and this was a considerable practical inconvenience. Finally, it was sometimes difficult to produce a state of true anaesthesia by the use of ether, because of 'intoxicated strugglings' and resistance to further inhalation. Neither was the perfect anaesthetic. The more thoughtful members of the profession in Britain soon realised, as one of them put it, that chloroform was 'both more powerful and more dangerous than ether'.[3]

To some extent the choice made depended principally on convenience and, in more senses than one, on taste. The Americans, who had pioneered ether, continued to use ether; the British, who had pioneered chloroform, continued to use chloroform. In Germany also chloroform was used, and so it was, on the whole, in France. But there was not a great deal of discussion.

This was probably because chloroform had indeed, as Simpson claimed, several obvious and immediate advantages over ether, and because, in a short time, controversy centred not on the question of relative merit but on the same doubts about the safety and propriety of anaesthesia using chloroform as had been expressed in 1847 regarding ether. Was pain in some way beneficial? Could narcotism induce convulsions? What were the concealed effects of chloroform on the patient? These were sensible questions but they were not answered because at least for the time being they could not be answered. In the 1940s and for long afterwards there was very little understanding of the functions of the central nervous system, and the neurophysiology of pain was a closed book. Even today we do not fully understand how narcosis comes about. We know that anaesthesia interrupts physiological functions, and that physiological functions are highly interrelated. Anaesthesia brings about biochemical and pathological changes in blood and tissues. The automatic nervous system is affected, hormone and enzyme activity is interfered with, metabolism is depressed, liver functions may be depressed, and changes occur in gaseous exchange in blood and tissues. Of all this Victorian medical science knew nothing, and suspected almost nothing. It is also of extreme importance that the manner of induction and depth of anaesthesia may cause oxygen shortage, carbon dioxide excess, and respiratory obstruction, while the environmental temperature and state of mind of the patient can have a profound influence on the biochemical changes. Of this the Victorian surgeons became in the course of time to some degree aware.

It follows that discussion of the physiological effects of chloroform was groping, limited, and often unsound. Few writers ventured upon the subject. One of the first was John Snow who, early in 1847, was already establishing himself as a leading authority on the induction of anaesthesia, having secured, with Liston's support, a near-monopoly of 'the ether practice in London'. Snow was an Englishman — a fact which was to prove of considerable importance in the anaesthesia controversy — born in 1813, two years after Simpson. In the old way he became apprenticed to a surgeon, near Newcastle, and then studied at the Hunterian School of Medicine in London, taking his MRCS in 1838. In many respects he was almost the opposite of Simpson. Where Simpson was restless, noisy and impulsive, Snow was patient, quiet, indefatigable. He had qualities that Simpson had not, and that few have; a shrewd perception of facts, a capacity for the dispassionate sifting of evidence, a resolution for comprehensive enquiry. He was one of the small band of men who, in the first half of the nineteenth century, did original research in medicine. In 1841 he achieved some prominence when he read a paper to the Westminster Medical Society entitled *On Asphyxia and on the Resuscitation of New-born Children*. In 1843 he produced a paper on the action of the capillary vessels in aiding the circulation of the blood, and in 1844 he wrote on the kidneys in Bright's disease. Later, in 1849, he became famous with his path-breaking *On the Mode of Communication of Cholera*, an essay which along with his phenomenal success five years later in reducing the frightful mortality from cholera in the Broad Street area of Soho by cutting off the local water supply, demonstrated to an at first incredulous profession that cholera was predominantly a water-borne disease. His researches on this subject were later described as 'master-works of medical learning'. Selfless and unassuming, Snow was one of the greatest British medical scientists, perhaps the greatest of the first half of the nineteenth century; an age, it must be admitted, when outstanding talent and medical enquiry had only a very occasional connection. When he died in 1858 the *Lancet* described him as easily the outstanding physician of all the physicians of his day.

Snow had become interested in anaesthesia before the discovery of chloroform, and early in 1847 he read a paper to the Westminster Medical Society in which he argued that the vapour of ether did not produce, as many thought, a kind of asphyxia by excluding oxygen from the lungs, but altered the composition of the blood so as to reduce to a minimum the oxidation of nervous and other tissues. This he restated more fully in 1851:

> Chloroform, ether, and similar substances, when present in the blood in certain quantities, have the effect of limiting those combinations between the oxygen of the arterial blood and the tissues of the body which are essential to sensation, volition, and, in short, all animal functions. The substances modify, and in larger quantities arrest, the animal functions, in the same way, and by the same power, that they modify and arrest combustion . . . when they are mixed in certain quantities with the atmospheric air.[4]

According to his biographer, Snow thought this

> the best observation he had ever made. Placing a taper, during one of our experiments, in a bottle through which chloroform vapour was diffused, and watching the declining flame, he once said, 'there, now, is all that occurs in narcotism; but to submit the candle to the action of the narcotic without extinguishing it altogether, you must neither expose it to too much vapour at once, nor subject it to the vapour too long; and this is all you can provide against in submitting a man to the same influence. I could illustrate all the meaning of this great practical discovery on a farthing candle, but I fear the experiment would be thought rather commonplace.'[5]

Another author who speculated on the subject was a rising young obstetrician, Tyler Smith. Tyler Smith was what the Victorians rejoiced to call 'a self-made man'. His early education was scanty, but in his native city of Bristol he acquired a medical training and a determination to make his fortune in London, where he arrived in 1840. He was without influence or connections, and to begin with depended largely on writing. He first came to prominence with a series of lectures on obstetrics published in the *Lancet* in 1847 and 1848. These were written at a time when he could have had little practical experience, but they formed the basis of his *Manual of Obstetrics* which became and for long remained the most popular English text-book on midwifery. Just before the publication of his lectures, in the spring of 1847, Tyler Smith gave a single lecture in which he treated the anaesthesia question both as a physiologist and as an obstetrician. 'Etherisation', he wrote, 'is chiefly a new condition of the nervous system'. This was a promising start, but he did a good deal less well with arguments about the cerebral faculties and the spinal marrow, 'the seat of the reflex function in its most extended signification'. His views, and those of his most enlightened contemporaries, are summed up in the following paragraph:

. . . there must be a special seat of pain, and special nerves for its propagation, from the periphery to the centre of painful sensation. . . it becomes a question whether ether affects the seat of pain, or the nerves which conduct to it. Mr Adams, of the London Hospital, made the ingenious suggestion that the blood was altered in etherisation, and that the altered blood paralysed the extremities of the nerves. Others have maintained that this altered condition of the blood depends on the imperfect inhalation of the ether, and partial asphyxia. We know that a writer of eminence on the nervous system is of opinion that the central seat of pain, with that of pleasurable sensations, and emotion, and respiration, is . . . the medulla oblongata, whilst its actual seat is in some part of the ganglionic system. Probably, under the full influence of ether, the whole of the nervous system concerned in the production and perception of pain is simultaneously affected.[6]

In short, various hypotheses were possible and several of those put forward by Tyler Smith are now perfectly archaic – 'a special seat of pain', 'special nerves for its propagation', 'imperfect inhalation' causing 'partial asphyxia'. Almost ten years later, medical opinion was in nearly the same state. Tyler Smith's ideas were repeated through the 1850s almost without alteration, and even those who had the greatest respect for John Snow – 'the most philosophical and skilful investigator of chloroform after its immortal discoverer, Dr Simpson' – were apt to regard his teaching, that an overdose caused paralysis of the heart through concentration of the poison in the blood, as competing on equal terms with notions of asphyxia and congestive apoplexy. Some speculations of the time were sensible; but for the most part they simply indicate the enormous ignorance of physiology which prevailed everywhere in the 1840s and 1850s.

This ignorance was a very serious matter, for patients had begun to die under chloroform. The first fatality occurred in England on 28 January 1848, only some ten weeks after the first use of chloroform. Hannah Greener, a healthy girl of 15 who had been operated on successfully under ether a few months before, was to have a toe-nail removed. The surgeon who gave the anaesthetic described the course of events as follows:

> She appeared to dread the operation, and fretted a good deal. . . The inhalation [the patient was seated in a chair] . . . was done from a handkerchief on which a teaspoonful of chloroform had been poured. . . In about a half a minute . . . finding her insensible, [I] requested Mr Lloyd to begin the operation. At the termination of the semi-lunar incision she gave a kick or twitch, which caused me to think the chloroform had not sufficient effect. I was proceeding to apply more to the handkerchief, when her lips, which had been previously of a good colour, became suddenly blanched, and she spluttered at the mouth, as if in epilepsy . . . I threw down the handkerchief, dashed cold water in her face, and gave her some internally, followed by brandy, without, however, the least effect. . . We laid her on the floor, opened a vein in her arm, and the jugular vein, but no blood flowed. The whole process of inhalation, operation, venesection, and death, could not, I should say, have occupied more than two minutes.[7]

This event aroused a great deal of interest and concern, both among the public and in medical circles. A post-mortem examination was carried out, and it was found that the lungs were 'in a very high state of congestion. . . The stomach was distended with food. . . The heart contained dark fluid blood in both cavities. . .' At the inquest the distinguished Newcastle surgeon, Sir John Fife, stated that 'in his opinion, the cause of death was the congestion of the lungs; and this congestion he was compelled to ascribe to the inhalation of chloroform. . . Of the power of chloroform to occasion such congestion no doubt can be entertained after the experiments of Mr Wakley and Dr Glover on animals. . .' Fife attributed the fatal result in Hannah Greener's case to

'some peculiarity in her constitution — not to be detected before-
hand — either in the lungs or in the nervous system'. And he added that
the surgeon who carried out the operation could not be held in any way
liable: 'No human foresight, no human knowledge, no degree of
science, could have forewarned any man against the use of chloroform
in this case.' This, if it was correct, was an extremely serious finding,
for it meant that no surgeon could be sure that the patient in his care
would not succumb, suddenly and unpredictably, to the administration
of chloroform.

The Greener case turned out to be only the first in a long series. A
few months later a 22-year-old man went to his 'surgeon-dentist' in
London to have some stumps of teeth removed and died under chloroform. One and a half drachms were given in an inhaler and the operator
claimed that he had previously administered chloroform or ether seven
or eight hundred times. On the other hand, the female servant who gave
evidence and who had herself been in charge of the inhaler explained
at the inquest that she usually administered chloroform to ladies while
the footman attended to the gentlemen unless he 'happened not to be
in the way'.[8] Casual administration of this sort soon declined. After a
fatality at Manchester Royal Infirmary in 1853 it was decided that in
future cases one person should administer 'this deadly though valuable
agent' while a second scrutinised the effects on the patient. But skilled
administrators sometimes had no better luck. A year later, in 1854,
death occurred in a case using Snow's inhaler, the drug being administered by an assistant-apothecary at St George's Hospital 'who is appointed to administer chloroform in all the surgical operations'.[9] It is
not possible to know how many deaths took place that were properly
attributable to chloroform. In the spring of 1852 Snow put the total
at 18. A year later an anonymous and unimpressive article in the *Lancet*
gave the figure at 42, but this was supposed to be for the whole world.
(The writer added that, if ether were included 'the total would have
been greatly increased'.[10]) It was frequently stated that many deaths
due to chloroform were hushed up or not reported. On the other hand,
some deaths said to be due to chloroform were probably the result of
haemorrhage, operative shock, or surgical miscalculation.

In any event, the exact number of deaths was not important. It soon
became clear that chloroform was a dangerous and could be a deadly
agent. Even two or three deaths per year would have made a strong impression; and the public did not forget that 'a very large audience,
amongst whom were not a few ladies', which had assembled at the
Royal Institution in January 1848 in order to learn about the relative

merits of ether and chloroform, had seen the lecturer chloroform a guinea pig, promising to revive it after a few minutes; at the end of which time the wretched animal was found to be dead. 'Numerous have been the triumphant quotations of this experiment as a clear and indisputable proof of the extreme danger of this agent', wrote the *Lancet*.[11] And several years later Symes remarked that 'an impression was made upon the public which was not soon effaced'.[12]

It was quite impossible for the advocates of chloroform to ignore these warnings or the reactions that they produced; nor did they wish to do so. But in the absence of knowledge of how chloroform worked it was not obvious what arguments they could or should use. Simpson made some very sensible observations in connection with Hannah Greener's death. He had, he said, 'felt and repeatedly expressed surprise' that other deaths had not already occurred through 'want of caution' in administration; and he conceded that, 'if exhibited in too strong a dose, and given uninterruptedly for too great a length of time, [chloroform] would doubtless produce serious consequences and even death'. But his explanation of the Hannah Greener fatality was the most unsatisfactory that was made − perhaps the most unsatisfactory that was possible. She died, Simpson wrote, because she 'fell into a state of syncope' such as he had seen 'in a few cases'; cold water was poured into her mouth, immediately followed by brandy; she could not swallow these liquids, and was, in fact, no more able to breathe 'than it would have been possible to inspire if the whole head and face had been . . . submersed'. She was thus killed not by the chloroform but by the attempts to revive her, the post-mortem observations being 'all exactly those produced by simple asphyxia'.[13] This explanation found both support and opposition, Snow remarking, with characteristic restraint, that it 'seems improbable'. Significantly, this did not prevent Simpson from arguing a few months later, with far less plausibility, that a fatality in Aberdeen was another case of asphyxia, caused this time by the patient falling face down on to a wet towel.

John Snow offered a different explanation of the Greener case. He had always emphasised the dangers of faulty administration and especially the risk of inducing a state of deep anaesthesia (what he called 'a snoring sleep') with rapidity, 'lest the narcotism should proceed a degree further on account of the cumulative property of the vapour after it is discontinued'.[14] His explanation of the death of Hannah Greener was along these lines. His reasoning was far more convincing than Simpson's, and it also cast doubt on the official view that some undiscoverable peculiarity in the patient had been the cause of death.

'My view of the matter', Snow wrote,

> holds out more hope for the future. I look on the result as only what
> was to be apprehended from the over-rapid action of chloroform
> when administered on a handkerchief. . . I have observed that the
> effects of the vapour may accumulate for about twenty seconds
> after the inhalation is discontinued, and this accumulation will be
> the more formidable in proportion to the quantity of vapour that
> is being inhaled at the moment, and the velocity with which the
> symptoms were being induced. . . Now, in the case under consider-
> ation, when the girl had inhaled for about half a minute, there was
> rigidity of the arm [indicating considerable anaesthesia] . . . suppos-
> ing that the cloth was removed at that very instant . . . if the vapour
> was inhaled of the same strength during the thirty seconds, its
> effects might increase at the same pace for twenty seconds longer;
> and at the end of fifty seconds from the commencement she would
> be [in a state] in which the respiratory movements are more or less
> paralysed, and become difficult, feeble, or irregular.[15]

He pointed out that the alarming symptoms had appeared 'after the
cloth with chloroform was removed from the patient's face'; narcotism
had then proceeded without further inhalation of chloroform to the
final stage of total cessation of respiration. Snow was anxious to
emphasise this danger. Simpson himself, he observed, had recorded
having seen 'in a few cases such a blanched state of the lips and features [as in the Greener case] come on, under the use of very powerful and deep doses of chloroform, simulating syncope, and with the
respiration temporarily suspended'. But the symptoms, according to
Simpson, 'rapidly disappeared' if the chloroformed napkin was removed and the patient let alone. Snow did not think that this was
good enough. Assuming that these were cases under Simpson's own
supervision, he wrote, 'this makes the danger still more evident; for
if anyone could prevent his patient from getting into a state which cannot be looked on otherwise than as one of imminent peril, it would be
the authority who introduced the agent, and recommended this method
of its administration'. His point was a strong one, and it linked with his
conviction (shared by the Scottish school) that safety lay in attending
to the respiration rather than the pulse — 'the respiration ceases, while
the circulation is still vigorous; [patients] die, in fact, as if by asphyxia'.
  Confused debate about who or what killed Hannah Green and
other early victims did not help very much towards a general under-

standing of the problem. In the mid-1850s it was still widely maintained that 'the whole matter rests . . . on idiosyncracies'[16] and that
no progress towards understanding had been made. But this was not
the case. Careful and correct administration was the secret of using
chloroform, and this was emphasised by several writers almost from
the beginning.

When Simpson announced the discovery of chloroform anaesthesia
he linked it with and restated the rules for the administration of ether
which he had published in September 1847. These were

(1) 'absolute quietude and freedom from mental excitement, both
during the induction of etherisation, and during recovery from it';
(2) 'the primary stage of exhilaration should be entirely avoided, or
at least reduced to the shortest possible limit . . . a very common,
but certainly a very unpardonable error, being to exhibit an imperfect and exciting, instead of perfect and narcotising dose of the
vapour'; (3) 'determining to avoid the commencement of the operation itself until . . . the patient is . . . thoroughly and indubitably
soporised by it'.[17]

Even today, this advice could hardly be improved upon. We know
now, as Simpson did not, that excitement causes physiological changes
that react with chloroform in a possibly highly dangerous manner; that
during the stage of light anaesthesia the patient is at risk; that it is
dangerous to stimulate in any way a patient who is not fully anaesthetised. It is precisely these dangers that Simpson's rules avoid, if possible.
Simpson also explained the importance of using correctly a cloth, with
fluid on it, held over the patient's face with the hand of the administrator held between cloth and face so as to admit air. These points he constantly repeated. Yet in 1860 he noted how he had 'often feared lest
the lives of patients should be sacrificed by the careless manner in
which, in particular, students and young practitioners sometimes
employ the damp folded cloth. . .'[18] Simpson's rules were developed
and slightly modified over the years, and similar rules, involving the
use of an inhaler, were developed in England by Snow and others. They
were constantly reiterated and emphasised by all those who advocated
chloroform anaesthesia. Yet an enormous amount of discussion took
place as if the question was simply one of using or not using chloroform.

At last, in 1855, the matter was put to the profession with exceptional clarity when Lister wrote out and the *Lancet* published Syme's

winter course of 22 lectures in surgery. In the second of these lectures Syme raised the question why chloroform produced different results in different cases. Fatalities kept occurring: yet for seven years chloroform 'has been almost daily given here [and] we have not had a fatal case'. The explanation, said Syme, had to be either that the chloroform used was different in different cases, or that the mode of administration was different, or that the patients in question were significantly different. This completely and correctly stated the problem, and exposed the illogicality of focusing attention exclusively on patient peculiarities, real or imagined.

All of what Syme went on to say had already been understood and explained by other workers. On the first point he observed that it had been well known for several years that chloroform varied a good deal in quality, and that only the purest form should be used in anaesthesia. This was certainly important. Badly prepared chloroform may contain phosgene, which has been used as a poison gas in warfare. It is also the case that unless stored in air-tight containers away from heat and light, oxidation to phosgene may occur. It is thus quite likely that some of the bad results experienced in the early years of chloroform anaesthesia were due to impurities in the drug – it was foolish to talk as if in all cases the substance inhaled was the same. As regards patient peculiarities, Syme's comment was that whereas in London great care was taken to administer chloroform only to patients free from chest affections, especially cardiac derangements, 'here we never ask questions as to the state of the heart or constitution of the patients'. Only the previous week, Syme stated, he had operated on a patient who had been advised in London that any operation would certainly kill him; 'I performed the operation under chloroform; and the first thing he did on waking was to ask for a cigar'. The most important point, however, was the mode of administration. Once more it was explained that Scots practice was to pour chloroform on a large porous surface such as a folded towel or a handkerchief, placing this over the mouth and nostrils so that the patient could breathe air as well as chloroform; and, because the effects should be produced as rapidly as possible,

we do not stint the quantity of chloroform. Then – and this is the most important point – we are guided as to the effect, not by the circulation, but entirely by the respiration; you never see anybody here with his finger on the pulse while chloroform is given. So soon as the breathing becomes stentorous we cease the administration;

from what I have learned, it is sometimes pushed further elsewhere, but this we consider in the highest degree dangerous. Attention to the tongue is another part which we find of great consequence. When respiration becomes difficult, or ceases, we open the mouth, seize the tip of the tongue with artery-forceps, and pull it well forward; and there can be little doubt that death would have occurred in some cases if it had not been for the use of this expedient.

You observe that in this matter I am very far from taking credit to myself; all that I have done has been to follow the example of Dr Simpson, and all that I would say respecting our brethren in London is, that they have not been so fortunate as to get into the right way in the first instance, and I would urge upon them to banish all previous notions, and to keep in view the essential points to which I have alluded.[19]

The tribute to Simpson is a generous one. But the reader can hardly fail to notice a certain patronising tone towards the unenlightened in London,
In the matter of chloroform — its use, properties, limitations, administration and everything else about it — there was, indeed, little love lost between London and Edinburgh. And Syme, of all men, was in a peculiarly good position to enjoy himself in this conflict, and to twist tails in London when the opportunity arose. In 1848, when already a very distinguished operator, Syme had been appointed Professor of Clinical Surgery at University College. This appointment made the *Lancet* very angry. It expressed 'disgust and indignation' that University College ('woefully misgoverned') had 'imported from Scotland a gentleman named Syme' to be Professor of Surgery, as if there were not many equally or better qualified men in London and the rest of England.

When *Scotchmen* have any good offices to give away in Scotland, do *they* send to London for persons to occupy the vacant posts? No indeed! Journeys of such a character are only made from North to South, and not from South to North.[20]

It was all due, the *Lancet* thundered, 'to the Scottish influence which prevails in the Council and Medical Faculty'. Syme was not made welcome in London, and he returned to Scotland after a few months. Now, in 1855, his was the longest series of lectures ever to be published in the *Lancet,* and when publication was complete the *Lancet* wrote, 'Of the surgical value of these contributions . . . there has been but one opinion in this country'.[21] Syme's position was unassailable. He was probably, by this time, the most distinguished surgeon in Europe. Before he died 15 years later he had administered chloroform in upwards of 5,000 cases without losing a single patient. His lectures reflect a mind exceptionally clear and orderly; that of a man calm, knowledgeable, practical, sensible, full of judgment.

John Snow replied to Syme's statement of principles. Like Syme, he also had administered chloroform in several thousand cases without losing a single patient, and he thus wrote with equal authority. He emphasised, as he had always done, the dangers of administering chloroform 'in a very insufficient state of dilution', causing sudden arrest of the action of the heart. He criticised methods of administration which, on Syme's own admission, caused breathing to become difficult or to cease; adding pointedly that in King's College 'the breathing of the patient never becomes difficult, or ceases, and it has never been necessary to pull out the tongue with the artery forceps'. On one or two minor points Snow and many of his colleagues did not agree. He denied, for example, that there was any particular danger in giving chloroform to a patient in a sitting position. He did not admit that fear ('an affection of the mind') could in any way combine with the effects of chloroform to increase danger to the patient. But on the basic principles of chloroform anaesthetic Snow agreed with Syme and Simpson. He also agreed with Syme that organic disease, even fatty degeneration of the heart, was not an impediment to the use of chloroform. And he never accepted the view ('popular with some administrators because it appeared to provide a ready explanation of otherwise inexplicable death in healthy subjects'[22]) that some untraceable idiosyncrasy of the patient could be a cause of death.

Snow did not approve, however, of the Scots mode of administration. From the beginning, chloroform was administered in England by means of an inhaler. These inhalers were continuously developed, and Snow himself designed one that was particularly successful and widely used. The advantage of an inhaler was that the absorption of chloroform into the lungs could be exactly determined and controlled; although, as Snow himself ruefully admitted, 'many persons allow an apparatus to get out of order, or they are too careless to consider the express purpose for which it was contrived'.[23] In Scotland, on the other hand, chloroform was invariably administered on a cloth or handkerchief. This method was simple, easy, cheap, and, in the view of Englishmen, dangerous. But it persisted. When in 1877 Lister came from Glasgow to London as Professor of Surgery at King's College he raised many eyebrows when he proceeded to anaesthetise his patients using some drops of chloroform on a handkerchief.

In spite of these differences of opinion and practice, it must have been clear to the entire profession by 1855 — what should have been understood at least five years earlier — that chloroform anaesthesis could be carried out with almost complete safety. On the other hand, it must also have been clear that knowledge of the action of drugs was extremely rudimentary, and several researchers rightly warned that there might be serious dangers in setting up processes that no one understood. The French, in particular, tended to take this line. Magendie, the most eminent French physiologist of the day, had observed as early as 1847 that 'intoxication caused by sulphuric ether' (and he might have added, or by any other drug) was 'little understood', and that only when it was thoroughly understood 'could one safely, and with a clear conscience, apply it to man'.[24] The work of Snow and others in the late 1840s and the 1850s was designed to extend knowledge of narcosis as far as possible, but ignorance and risks remained. Thus the question that faced the profession — and the public, although they seem to have expressed their views, effectively no doubt, solely as individual patients — was whether chloroform anaesthesia was worth the risk.

This question first arose in surgery. Sir John Fife, in his report on the Greener fatality, had emphasised that he himself would insist upon taking chloroform in any operation involving much pain, and that he would continue to administer it even 'with the fatal result in the present instance staring him in the face'. He was convinced, he said, that the danger was 'comparatively small'. But not all surgeons were so categoric, and several specific objections were raised. One was that pain acts as 'the natural incentive to reparative action', that the prevention of pain would 'produce very serious depressing effects upon the nervous system' and seriously reduce the patient's powers of recovery. This argument, which was voiced by some of the most distinguished English surgeons of the day, was one for which no evidence whatever was produced, nor could be produced. It was also argued that to suspend sensation 'is to set at nought the ordinances of nature'. But the answer to this was that human sensibilities are given to avoid pain, not to promote it, and that excess pain has no salutary effect on character. Another objection to the use of chloroform in surgery was that pain might serve a useful purpose — the groans and cries of the patient might in some cases be 'an useful guide to the surgeon'. What might be called the classic statement of this objection was made by a Dr Coulson, addressing the Medical Society of London as late as October 1855. A 'case of lithotrity', he said,

> may be mentioned. It must be confessed that it would be an advant-age if chloroform could be employed. . . Yet when the nature of this delicate operation is considered, carried on, as it were, in the dark, and when it is further borne in mind that the operator should be fully aware of every step he is taking; in an organ completely removed from his sight, it cannot be expedient to render the patient insensible, and thus lose the aid which his feelings afford. . . A case in point occurred in a public hospital before the introduction of crushing, at a time when the perforator alone was employed. Notwithstanding the cries of the patient, the surgeon went on using the perforator in a most industrious manner. The bystanders feared something wrong, but the surgeon appealed to the sound of a metal-lic body striking against stone, as a proof that the calculus was actually seized, and undergoing the process of perforation. In a few seconds the cries of the patient became more violent; blood issued abundantly from the urethra. The bystanders now interfered, and pointed out to the surgeon, that the noise which he had heard was produced by the external end of the perforator striking against the seals of his watch-chain. The operation was suspended, and the patient's life saved; but had he been insensible, there is no saying what mischief might not have been inflicted, for the calculus was not between the blades of the instrument.[25]

The reaction of the audience to this alarming revelation of surgical incompetence is not recorded. Clearly, it was not a good case to quote against the use of chloroform; and in any case arguments of this kind were seldom put forward — except in obstetrics — after the early years.

It was also maintained that anaesthesia, while it prevented the patient from experiencing pain, did nothing to reduce the shock of the injury that was inflicted on the physical structure. This led to desultory discussion as to the nature of and connection between shock and pain; but this discussion was inevitably fruitless, because no one understood the physiology of either pain or shock, and in any case there was no argument against the use of chloroform unless it could be shown that the removal of pain actually increased operative shock; and this could not be shown. Simpson, indeed, tried to produce figures implying the reverse, namely, that chloroform anaesthesia tended to reduce the very high mortality resulting from operations. He wrote to every hospital in Britain, and to Paris, asking for returns of the operations carried out. Returns from almost 50 hospitals were received, and Simpson then tried to compare the results obtained in hospitals where anaesthetics were used with results where they were not. Selecting for special emphasis amputation of the thigh as perhaps the most dangerous operation common in surgery — the post-operational death rate in this class of case was stated by Syme in 1845 to be not less than 60 to 70 per cent — Simpson sought to show that under anaesthesia the death rate was reduced to 25 per cent. He admitted that the number of operations with anaesthesia that he had collected — 145 in total — was somewhat small from a statistical point of view, and because his statistics came from various parts of England, Scotland, and Ireland, as well as from Paris, it is obvious that there must be great doubt about the comparability of the cases. But combined with some forceful argument in a long paper entitled *Does anaesthesia increase or decrease the mortality attendant upon surgical operations?*, published in April 1848, these statistics served their purpose, and opposition on this score began to fade. The fatality at Newcastle, 'trumpeted a good deal in the newspapers', made some surgeons as well as patients hesitate. Doubt continued even to the mid-1850s, when it was not uncommon to argue that the risk of using chloroform should be avoided except in serious or unusually painful operations. But the advantages, both for surgeon and patient, were too great to be given up. Chloroform, helped us, as well as itself encouraging, the development of skill in surgery, transformed the scene. F.J. Grant, speaking in London in 1872, put the position as follows:

The old operators — ignorant often of anatomy, and always of pathology — are described as 'agitated, trembling, miserable, hesitating in the midst of difficulties, turning round to their friends for that support which should come from within, feeling in the wound for things which they did not understand, holding consultations amid the cries of the patient, or even retiring to consult about his case, while he lay bleeding, in great pain and awful expectation'. Nowadays, this picture is commonly reversed: witness the calm composure of the surgeon and the placid sleep of the patient.[26]

Within four years of its introduction chloroform had been used with success in many score of operational cases at St Bartholomew's alone.

There took place, indeed, a sudden and substantial increase in the number of operations — an 'operating mania', contemporaries called it. Ovarian tumours, it was said, were removed without good reason (not always successfully), and the head of the thigh was submitted to the knife and the saw 'with as much nonchalance as though it were being removed from the dead body in the dissecting room'.[27] This, it was declared, was mostly the work of younger surgeons, 'promising young men' who, with the help of chloroform, began 'to carve their way into practice'. Their elders were inclined to be shocked, and some patients lost their lives; but more, and earlier, operations undoubtedly reduced illness and suffering and usually prolonged useful life.

The relative ease with which chloroform triumphed in operative surgery contrasts sharply with the strenuous and prolonged opposition it met with in midwifery. This mattered a great deal, because while midwifery is only one of the many branches of medicine, it is one which vitally affects a very large percentage of the population every year. In the middle of the nineteenth century approximately 700,000 births took place in Great Britain annually. The death rate among mothers was high — almost certainly over one in every 200 cases. Surgical operations, on the other hand, prior to the introduction of anaesthesia, probably did not exceed a few thousand per annum. The figures are doubtful. But at the very least, the yearly number of ob-stetric cases was fifty-fold, and was more probably nearer a hundred-fold, the yearly number of surgical cases when the fight for anaesthesia began. As for the experience of giving birth, this varied, by our anaes-thetic and hygienic standards, from bad to almost indescribably dread-ful. One of the best-known obstetricians in Germany described the last stage of natural labour in the following words:

> the pains . . . are still more severe, painful, and enduring; return after a short interval, and take a far greater effect upon the patient than those of the previous stage. Their severity increases so much the more from the additional suffering arising from the continually increasing distension of the external parts. . . The bearing down becomes more continued, and there is not unfrequently vomiting. The patient quivers and trembles all over. Her face is flushed, and, with the rest of the body, is bathed in perspiration. Her looks are staring and wild; the features alter so much that they can scarcely be recognised. Her impatience rises to its maximum with loud crying and wailing, and frequently expressions which, even with sensible, high principled women, border close upon insanity.[28]

Suffering might not be so severe in the case of second and subsequent births. On the other hand, things might go wrong. One Sunday
evening in 1847 a Dr Moore, living in Hackney Road, London, received
an urgent message requesting him to visit immediately 'a lady residing
at Dalston'. Reaching the house, he found

a tall, powerful woman, very robust — about forty years of age —
forcibly held in the bed by several persons. . . Two doctors previously summoned had been so furiously assaulted, that they had
left, and declined to have anything to do with the case.

The midwife, in a supercilious, half-drunken, ignorant manner, was
loud in her protest against the intrusion of a medical man, asserting
that she knew her business, and did not want any interference; for
if the people would hold the patient, she could and would deliver
her without any doctor, so much better than any of them.

The midwife had been fetched on Saturday at four p.m. as the
patient had labour pains of tolerable strength, and at short intervals.
The midwife, upon examination, ruptured the membranes, and
ordered a strong glass of brandy and water to be made hot, into
which she placed a quantity of brown powder (ergot!) and this she
repeated several times in the course of the night, at the same time
taking herself some brandy. The pains, from being intermittent,
became violent and continuous, but seemingly without satisfactory
progress, until about six a.m.; when the midwife assured all around,
that although the patient was becoming delirious there was no
danger, and that she should administer something that would give
the patient some sleep for a few hours, when she would herself
return, to get over the case safely. She then gave some drops (tincture of opium), and left; but the patient growing more delirious,
the midwife being again fetched, administered more laudanum at
various intervals, and the patient grew more and more violent. . .

Finding the patient furiously delirious on the accession of the
pains, which were almost continuous, but feeble; and finding, after
considerable resistance, the pulse beating like a sledge-hammer,
at 100, the conjunctivae gorged, pupils dilated, and face flushed
and of a dull crimson hue; I determined to abstract blood (a proceeding loudly denounced by the midwife) to thirty ounces. I then
applied some evaporating lotion to the head, and after some time it

produced a state of partial tranquility.

Dr Moore then 'proceeded to an examination per vaginam, the patient screaming out the moment I touched her, from excessive tenderness. I found the external and internal labia enormously swollen, hot and dry, not the slightest secretion (a hand protruding between), the bladder distended, and the rectum loaded with faeces.' He therefore 'drew off two pints of high-coloured turbid urine', but was not allowed to leave 'to get my enema apparatus, the door being locked, as they feared I should perhaps leave them in the lurch, as the other gentlemen had done'. So three enemata were sent for and administered (unloading the bowel 'of an enormous quantity of faeces and flatus') and the patient calmed down although showing no diminution of the swelling and no tendency to secretion. Warm water was applied, and 40 drops of chloroform administered upon a sponge. 'In less than one minute the patient became perfectly tractable.' She was kept under 'by putting 20 drops upon the sponge from time to time' and a child was shortly delivered 'which is alive, and likely to live'.[29] Not all women were so fortunate as in this case, apart from the chloroform, seemingly administered as a last resort. Another physician in London attended a case in which

. . . the head advanced and receded slightly [in the cavity of the pelvis] at each pain; the vagina was dry and of a stinging heat; the pains were slight, occurring every two minutes, and apparently cut short by the screams and disordered efforts and motions of the patient. The latter was in a state of frantic agitation, screaming and plunging in every direction as soon as the pains came on. . . The skin was hot and dry; the pulse full, 120; the eyes bloodshot, the face injected; the tongue white, but moist. Had chloroform not been available I should certainly have felt myself called upon to take fifteen or twenty ounces of blood from the arm, in order to remove the general congestion, and to allay the irritability of the nervous system.[30]

After the administration of chloroform the pulse fell to 90, the pains became bearable, and the child was still-born. Ordeals like these might last for as long as 40 or 50 hours; there are statements of labour, 'laborious labour', lasting for as long as 80 and 90 hours. To make matters worse, very severe and protracted labour was apt to end in instrumental delivery, very possibly occasioning the death of the child, and sometimes of the mother as well. And there was always, of course, the danger that puerperal fever would set in a day or two later.

These were the kind of conditions that Simpson must have had in mind when he set off on his campaign to convince the profession that chloroform anaesthesia ought to be used in child-birth. What he had to show was that chloroform was, if not safe, at any rate safe enough; and that if it was safe enough it should be used. His line of argument on the first of these points tended to be that any drug could be dangerous if mishandled, that accidents were caused not by chloroform but by its incompetent administration. Responding to Professor Meigs of Philadelphia, a very well-known American obstetrician, Simpson wrote as follows:

I do believe that if improperly and incautiously given, and in some rare idiosyncrasies, ether and chloroform may prove injurious or even fatal — just as opium, calomel, and every other powerful remedy and strong drug will occasionally do. Drinking cold water itself will sometimes produce death.

He pointed out that according to the Registrar General 242 deaths had occurred in 1844 as a result of poisons, all of which had been prescribed as medicinal; if chloroform were to be prohibited, why, he asked, should not all these other poisons be prohibited also? Many fatalities he attributed to the use of impure chloroform. Struggling, choking and death under chloroform were almost always the result, he reiterated again and again, either of bad administration or of impurities in the drug. To these two causes he later added a third, fear. Nervous, apprehensive or excited patients might be killed by their own emotion, he declared, but not by chloroform. As to the desirability of using chloroform — or ether — in childbirth as well as in surgery, Simpson never had any doubt at all, and he lost no opportunity to press his views. He was resolved to use these anaesthetics and to lessen pain, not next year nor next month but now, and his resolution and humanity made his contribution to the debate on anaesthesia extremely important, if scientifically undistinguished.

Almost from the date that ether anaesthesia became known, Simpson used ether in childbirth. From early in 1847, he wrote, he was using ether 'with few and rare exceptions, in every case of labour that I have attended'[31] and in November of that year he told his class that in several deliveries 'he had continued the sleep for eight and ten hours with perfect comfort and safety to the patient'.[32] As early as February 1847 he published a paper which shows how, from the very start, he adopted a determined, crusading, indeed aggressive attitude.

> The question which I have been repeatedly asked is this — will we ever be 'justified' in using the vapour of ether to assuage the pains of natural labour? Now, if experience betimes goes fully to prove to us the safety with which ether may, under proper precautions and management, be employed in the course of parturition, then, looking to the facts of the case, and considering the amount of pain usually endured, I believe that the question will require to be quite changed in its character. For, instead of determining in relation to it whether we shall be 'justified' in using this agent under the circumstances named, it will become, on the other hand, necessary to determine whether on any grounds, moral or medical, a professional man could deem himself 'justified' in withholding and *not* using any such safe means (as we at present pre-suppose this to be), provided he had the power by it of assuaging the pangs and anguish of the last stage of natural labour, and thus counteracting what Velpeau describes as 'those piercing cries, that agitation so lively, those excessive efforts, those inexpressible agonies, and those pains apparently intolerable', which accompany the termination of natural parturition in the human mother.[33]

This is an emphatic but not an unqualified statement. It refers only to the use of anaesthesia in the last stage of labour, there is a careful reference to the need for further experience to prove the safety of the drug, and the need for 'proper precaution and management' is recognised. But the question of the 'justification' of using anaesthesia in natural labour had evidently already been raised. Nine months later, in November, Simpson published a small pamphlet entitled *Remarks on the Superinduction of Anaesthesia in Natural and Morbid Parturition*. The tone of this pamphlet is quite different from that of the February essay. Instead of a calm statement of the advantages of anaesthesia it is an angry attack on the conservatism of the medical profession.

> All of us, I most sincerely believe, are called upon to employ it [anaesthesia] by every principle of true humanity, as well as by every principle of true religion. Medical men may oppose for a time the superinduction of anaesthesia in parturition, but they

will oppose it in vain; for certainly our patients themselves will force the use of it upon the profession. The whole question is, even now, one merely of time. It is not − Shall the practice come to be generally adopted? but, When shall it come to be generally adopted? Of course, it will meet from various quarters with all due and determinate opposition. Medical men will, no doubt, earnestly argue that their established medical opinions and medical practices should not be harshly interfered with by any violent innovations of doctrine regarding the non-necessity and non-propriety of maternal suffering. They will insist on mothers continuing to endure, in all their primitive intensity, all the agonies of childbirth, as a proper sacrifice to the conservatism of the doctrine of the desirability of pain. They will perhaps attempt to frighten their patients into the medical propriety of this sacrifice of their feelings; and some may be found who will unscrupulously ascribe to the new agencies any misadventures, from any causes whatever, that may happen to occur in practice. But husbands will scarcely permit the suffering of their wives to be perpetuated merely in order that the tranquility of this or that medical dogma be not rudely disturbed. Women themselves will betimes rebel against enduring the usual tortures and miseries of child-birth, merely to subserve the caprice of their medical attendants. And I more than doubt if any physician is really justified, on any grounds, medical or moral, in deliberately desiring and asking his patients to shriek and writhe on in their agonies for a few months, or a few years longer, in order that, by doing so, they may defer to his professional apathy, or pander to his professional prejudices.

This was far more a biting criticism of fellow practitioners than a defence of anaesthesia in child-birth, and it was not calculated to conciliate − any more than it was sufficient to silence − the opposition. But what was the opposition? Who were these 'medical men' whose arguments and behaviour, either already encountered or merely anticipated, Simpson so vehemently condemned?

The first in point of time, and also one of the most prominent, was Tyler Smith, latterly obstetric physician and lecturer on obstetrics at St Mary's Hospital, London. In March 1847, when only Simpson and Dubois had published on the use of ether in midwifery, Tyler Smith gave a lecture, already referred to in this chapter, entitled 'On the Utility and Safety of the Inhalation of Ether in Obstetric Practice'.[34] The lecture as published is about 4,000 words in length, far more substantial than most contributions to the *Lancet*. Tyler Smith may be said to approach the question from a 'scientific', a practical, and a 'moral' point of view. No indication is given that the author himself had ever exhibited ether.

Tyler Smith begins by acknowledging that the removal of pain is, in itself, good. But what other effects does ether produce? Etherisation being 'a new condition of the nervous system', there are effects on sensation, volition and emotion. All of these help in parturition. Volition aids some efforts; and in the final pains of labour, which admittedly are not controlled by the will, intense pain makes the patient cry out, an action which 'opens the glottis, takes away all expiratory pressure, and leaves the uterus acting alone. So, in the last stage of labour, upon the mingled agony and exertion of which obstetricians have exhausted their descriptive powers, pain and its attendant emotion play a benign and salutary part.' Secondly, there is the argument that labour is a species of shock, in which pain is an element. Shock depresses the system, but pain 'sometimes acts as a stimulant, and as such is probably salutary rather than prejudicial'. Emotion is another element in shock. 'Many parturient women', says Tyler Smith, 'are destroyed, directly or indirectly, by emotion alone, and so are many surgical patients'. This looks like an argument in favour of anaesthesia; but no deduction is drawn.

So far the weight of the argument is very much against anaesthesia, although not emotionally so, but the two main points are still to be made. The first of these involves Tyler Smith's supposedly scientific account of the functioning of the nervous system. Shock, he says, 'in its true nature' affects the spinal marrow and the ganglionic system even more than the brain. Labour is the result of, or is connected with, 'utero-spinal excitement'. Ether affects first the cerebral faculties and then the spinal marrow, tending to cause, as a result, 'spasmodic twitchings, or even general convulsions'. But parturient women have in any case 'a tendency to convulsions'. It is therefore 'improper to resort, without very grave reason, to the use of an agent so capable of adding to the utero-spinal excitement of labour, a new and a direct stimulant [sic] of the organ concerned in convulsions'. This pseudo-science probably carried a good deal of weight in the 1840s and 1850s. Tyler Smith had, of course, no means of knowing what connections existed, if any, between the spinal marrow, the ganglionic system and the brain on the one hand and either ether or convulsions on the other. Utero-spinal excitement was a phenomenon that existed solely in his imagination. But he had noted (correctly) that uterine contractions were not necessarily affected by ether, and he supposed that shock, possibly leading to convulsions, might occur even in the absence of sensibility. Given that neither he nor anyone else knew what shock consisted of, the argument appeared not unreasonable. It forms the central core of Tyler Smith's case against anaesthesia, and is the longest part of his paper.

Finally, he touched on an aspect of etherisation that greatly shocked contemporaries. This was 'the occasional incitement of the sexual passion in patients under the influence of ether'. Pain, as he put it, was 'metamorphosed into its antithesis'.

> I may venture to say, that to the women of this country the bare possibility of having feelings of such a kind excited and manifested in outward uncontrollable actions, would be more shocking even to anticipate, than the endurance of the last extremity of physical pain. I am only surprised that the distinguished French obstetrician [Dubois] should not have made some observation of this kind.

The observed fact, and the judgment regarding British (or did he mean English?) female preference, occupy about one-fifth of the whole essay.

With all these arguments at his command, Tyler Smith had no difficulty in deciding against anaesthesia in obstetrics. Even in surgery it was of doubtful benefit. 'There has been a general rush towards the operating room', he observed, 'such as the world has never before witnessed'. But fatalities inevitably take place because of the idiosyncracies of patients — the plea that faulty administration is the source of trouble cannot be accepted. In obstetrics the matter is even clearer. Etherisation does not diminish shock and it increases the risk of puerperal convulsions; and again, it may accidentally and of itself kill the patient. It will, therefore, 'be rarely, if ever, used in difficult parturition or obstetric operations, and certainly never in natural labour'. Science must 'continue her search after some certain and available relief from physical pain'.

Tyler Smith's is a thoughtful critique. It is based, evidently, on no direct experience of anaesthesia. It is a genuine attempt at analysis, and uses some of the physiological ideas in vogue at the time. But the number of cases referred to is absolutely minimal, nothing is said about the purity or impurity of ether, and the argument that faulty administration could be a frequent source of trouble is dismissed without examination. Much is made of the alleged tendency for etherisation to bring on convulsions (for which there was very scant evidence;

Tyler Smith even quotes in this connection two cases listed by Dubois in which the mothers died not of convulsions but of puerperal fever), and although the tone of the essay is detached and unemotional it is quite clear that the 'sexual passion' argument was in his mind, of itself, decisive. Altogether, this essay is not untypical of medical argument at the time. It is scientific after a fashion; contains moral judgments of absolute conviction; and betrays no grasp whatever of the importance of collecting and carefully surveying available evidence. In the 1840s it was undoubtedly an acceptable statement of the case against anaesthesia.

A few weeks later the *Lancet* carried a short paper by Protheroe Smith, Assistant Teacher of Midwifery at St Bartholomew's Hospital, and a rising medical practitioner in the West End of London. This paper is in effect a reply to Tyler Smith, and is perhaps as sane, scientific and well argued as any paper then published on the subject. Protheroe Smith asks three questions: Is the abolition of pain in child-birth 'justifiable on Christian principles? as I have frequently been asked'; what are 'the *a priori* physiological probabilities' in inhaling ether? and what are 'the results of the cases in which ether has been tried'? This sets up the problem in a very clear way. He took the question of principle with the greatest seriousness (he was a man of marked Evangelical views), saying that if etherisation in child-birth was not justifiable on Christian principles 'all discussion of the other questions must be at once abandoned'. But 'why bear evils easily removable?' The pain of child-birth, like any other pain or physical ailment, was an evil to be removed if possible. Vaccination had been condemned when first introduced on the ground that 'the practice was a presumptuous contravention of the Divine will'. Now, he said, everyone accepts vaccination. If objections of this kind are to be made, they could be made 'with far more reason' to the practice of inducing premature labour,

> and still more strongly against destroying *in utero* a living foetus.
> Yet it is now universally admitted, that to risk the life of the mother
> by refraining from these operations, is not only unjustifiable but
> highly criminal.[35]

Having thus settled the question of principle, Protheroe Smith dealt briefly with the 'physiological probabilities'. He pointed out that pain depresses the spirits and is a large element (how large no one knows) in shock, and harmful effects can be avoided by controlling the dose and observing the symptoms. The remainder of the paper is a very careful,

factual description of three cases using ether, one requiring instrumental delivery. In each case there was great and immediate relief to
the patient, relaxation of the muscles, no diminution of uterine contractions, and no subsequent ill effects.

Protheroe Smith's paper, along with Simpson's two essays and the
lecture by Tyler Smith, were all published before the discovery of
chloroform anaesthesia. This discovery affected the debate in a number
of ways. For one thing, it very much intensified interest in the whole
subject of anaesthesia in child-birth. It was at once reported in every
medical journal and the *British and Foreign Medico-Chirurgical Review*
referred to it as 'a most important improvement'. But for another, it
made the name and personality of Simpson, conspicuously and un-
avoidably, a principal part of the whole affair.

Simpson was always an enthusiast for new ideas, and he throve on
conflict and controversy. It was not in his nature to await quietly the
triumph, however inevitable, of what he believed to be right. Also, he
knew how hard it often is to have new ideas accepted in medicine, or
for that matter in any other field. When, 'in the progress of the march
of knowledge and science', he wrote, old practices are challenged,
'human practices and prejudices ever rise up to argue for, and insist
upon, the continuance and safety of the past, and the total impolicy
and high peril of any attempted alteration'.[36] He was wont, in later
years, to impress upon his students this idea that anything new meets
with resistance. When the mail coach to London from Edinburgh cut
the time for the journey from twelve days to three, he told them,
travellers were advised to spend a night at York, 'as several who had
gone straight through were said to have died of apoplexy from the
rapidity of the motion'. Spectacles and the telescope, when they first
appeared, were branded by the Church as 'offsprings of man's wicked
mind' because they changed the natural appearance of things. Tea and
coffee were denounced as aphrodisiacs. The reception accorded to ether
and chloroform, said Simpson, was very similar. They were supposed on
their introduction to cause 'great moral and physical evils and injuries'
which, by and by, were found to be much the same as those caused by
tea and hackney coaches. One of Simpson's great advantages was his
knowledge of the past, and, unlike most of his opponents, he was as
capable of appealing to medical history as to current practice or the
Bible.

From the very beginning of etherisation Simpson resolved that the
use of anaesthesia in obstetrics should and must succeed; and he clearly
anticipated the kind of opposition usually encountered by any such

'great proposed change in practice'. His two early papers on the subject, already quoted, prove this. The discovery of chloroform anaesthesia strengthened his attitude. In the paper announcing his discovery he wrote, 'I have no doubt whatever that some years hence the practice [of using chloroform in child-birth] will be general. Obstetricians may oppose it, but I believe our patients themselves will force the use of it upon the profession.'[37] And he added in a footnote that he understood that few obstetricians in London used ether, and that a letter from Professor Montgomery informed him that in Dublin ether had never been used in child-birth. A few weeks later he returned to the attack. Was it right and proper to assuage or remove these awful pains of parturition 'beyond all description?' Such questions, he wrote, are often

> . . . complacently put by medical men. . . They are questions propounded with all imaginable gravity and seriousness by individuals who (in a mere abstract point of view) would, no doubt, strongly object to being considered as anxious to patronise and abet the continuance of pain, or traffic in the perpetuation of human sufferings of any kind.[38]

And he went on to allege that 'not one in twenty, perhaps not one in a hundred, of the physicians and surgeons of Great Britain' had, as yet, 'thought seriously upon the propriety of annulling the tortures attendant on human parturition'. He conceded that some physicians were ready to argue that pain was an advantage, even beneficial. But this doctrine was 'fundamentally unsound'. And he referred to his February pamphlet, already quoted, in which he had recorded his belief 'that we are, all of us, called upon to employ [anaesthesia] by every principle of true humanity, as well as by every principle of true religion'. This outburst, published only three weeks after the discovery of chloroform anaesthesia, drew the understandable retort that rational men could not 'thus be dragooned into adopting, in every case of natural labour, the use of a hazardous and doubtful agent'.[39]

Simpson's appeal was to the principles of 'true humanity' and 'true religion'. The medical advantages and disadvantages of chloroform he rarely discussed, and physiology never. That he avoided the latter topic was just as well, because nothing was to be gained through arguments depending on misconceived functions and contestable hypotheses. As to the clinical effects of anaesthesia, he was from the start convinced that facts and experience would win the day. The principles of true religion, on the other hand, had to be established. Religious objection

was raised, first in Scotland, to anaesthesia in child-birth. The Bible
said, 'In sorrow thou shalt bring forth children', and it followed that to
remove the sorrow or at least reduce it, was to contravene God's will.
This line of argument, contrary to what might be supposed, was not
particularly popular with the ministers of the church. In particular,
Dr Thomas Chalmers, leader of the newly created Free Church, a great
humanitarian and one of the most influential men in Scotland, counten-
anced the use of chloroform by witnessing operations performed with
its assistance in the Edinburgh Royal Infirmary and, when asked to deal
in a magazine article with the theological aspect of anaesthesia in child-
births refused on the ground that the question had no theological aspect
(Chalmers had been a professor of divinity) and he proceeded to advise
Miller, Simpson and their supporters to take no notice of the 'small
theologians' who wrote as if it had. But Simpson was never one to
ignore opponents and he entered into this aspect of the controversy
with evident relish. He never questioned that religious arguments were
appropriate; he never hesitated to use them himself; and he demolished
those of his opponents with a greater show of scholarship than they,
and better sense.

Was it decreed that in sorrow women should bring forth children?
Not at all; that is a mistranslation. To be well informed in these matters
is to know that

> . . . the Hebrew term which, in our English translation of the prime-
> val curse, is rendered 'sorrow' (Genesis, iii, 16), principally signifies
> the severe muscular *efforts* and *struggles* of which parturition – and
> more particularly human parturition – essentially consists; and does
> not specially signify the *feelings* or sensations of pain to which these
> muscular efforts or contractions give rise.[40]

Chloroform annuls the feelings and sensations; it leaves unchanged the
efforts and struggles to which alone the curse refers. Simpson's most
famous pamphlet on the ethico-religious aspects of anaesthesia was
entitled *Answer to the Religious Objection Advanced against the
Employment of Anaesthetic Agents in Midwifery and Surgery*. Ten
thousand copies were printed, and it was prefaced with two texts from
the New Testament: 'For every creature of God is good, and nothing to
be refused, if it be received with thanksgiving' (Tim. 4:4); and 'Therefore to him that knoweth to do good and doeth it not, to him it is
Sin' (Jas. 4:17).

In Scotland Simpson was rapidly triumphant, but in the summer of

1848 he received a letter from Protheroe Smith saying that in London 'the progress of anaesthetic midwifery is impeded by . . . groundless allegations as to its unscriptural character'. Simpson's draft reply to this letter — a little franker than the one he ultimately sent — states that to begin with many Edinburgh patients had 'strong religious scruples on the propriety of the practice'. Some consulted their minister; and one clergyman expressed the opinion that the use of chloroform in child-birth would 'harden society and rob God of the deep earnest cries which arise in time of trouble for help'. But religious opposition, Simpson wrote,

> has now entirely ceased among us, if we except an occasional remark on the point from some caustic old maid whose prospects of using chloroform are for ever passed, or a sneer from some antiquated lady who grieves and grudges that her daughters should not suffer as their mother was obliged to suffer before them.[41]

Then, after reiterating his argument that the primeval curse referred to muscular efforts and not to labour pains, Simpson went on to say that those who objected to the use of chloroform because it was contrary to

> . . . the object and end of the primeval curse upon woman, strangely forget, that the whole science and whole art and practice of midwifery is, in its essence and object, one continuous effort to mitigate and remove the effects of that curse. . . If, on religious grounds, your obstetric friends object to relieving entirely a woman of her worst pains, now that they have the means of doing so, they must on the very same grounds refuse to relieve her imperfectly and partially of these or any other parturient pains; they must, or at least ought to abstain in fact from all obstetric practices whatsoever; they should, in short, give up their present profession as a profession of sin.[42]

It is not recorded that anyone followed this advice. Instead, the religious objections were soon abandoned, and a large number of doctors adopted a compromise. Given only a moderate amount of suffering, they said, chloroform should not be used. But if there were pains 'of a severe, urgent and exhausting nature', then its use was admissible, or desirable, or even, perhaps, an imperative duty. Scenes 'of almost indescribable suffering and distress' should be converted into calmness and serenity. Extreme exhaustion, after all, was itself a danger. And yet, even those who argued in this way often sounded uneasy. They stressed that pain, extreme pain, and danger justified their actions. They did not deny, often very readily acknowledged, that there was an essential impropriety in exhibiting chloroform in midwifery.

> That every woman about to pass through the ordeal to which she is doomed by the laws of Nature, under the interesting circumstances of her becoming a mother, should henceforth be rendered insensible throughout the whole of the proceedings, is alike repulsive to good taste and sound judgment.[43]

And of course there was also the question of balancing 'natural' dangers to the mother against the danger created by using chloroform.

These and other doubts had been raised in Tyler Smith's 1847 paper. An additional argument was put forward in 1848 by G.T. Gream, Physician-Accoucheur to Queen Charlotte's Lying-in Hospital and one of the most successful and fashionable obstetricians working in the West End of London. He was also one of the most vocal but not quite the most unreasonable of the anti-anaesthesia school. Chloroform, according to Gream, did not accelerate labour; on the contrary, 'in one of the largest metropolitan hospitals where it has been employed, it has been found invariably to retard delivery'.[44] This was a serious matter, because it was generally (although not always) recognised that the longer the labour lasted the greater was the danger. Moreover, as Robert Barnes pointed out, a long labour was quite likely to end in delivery with instruments, which greatly increased the risk of a fatality. Barnes reckoned that in Great Britain delivery with instruments resulted in the death of the mother in one case in twenty and of the child oftener than one case in five. This was, therefore, 'a most fatal objection to the indiscriminate use of chloroform'.[45]

This argument is rather typical of the factual discussions that took place. Some, like Gream and Barnes, declared that chloroform lengthened labour, but others were equally emphatic that it did not — 'the action of the uterus is not interfered with', 'the natural process goes on with more regularity when not under the influence of the will of the patient'.[46] Contradictory statements appeared in successive weeks, sometimes in the same week. And although it was pointed out not once but twice in 1848, by two different doctors each working and speaking in London, that, as one of them put it, confusion arose 'for the want of an accurate description of the time and mode of exhibiting the agent in most of the published cases; for no doubt different results ensue from different doses, and from different modes of administration',[47] the main contestants continued to write and speak as if chloroform as such produced the results which they declared to have been found and verified – not necessarily by themselves.

The absence of incontrovertible, or at any rate of uncontested, evidence left the field open for endless asseveration, disputation, repetition. In 1848 and 1849 the *Lancet* carried four long contributions on the subject as well as reporting at considerable length three debates in the Westminster Medical Society, all quite inconclusive. Further similar offerings appeared in the early 1850s, the last considerable one in 1853. Because there was so much repetition, there is no need to indicate the substance and tone of more than two of these items.

G.T. Gream, as already mentioned, was an early opponent of chloroform anaesthesia in childbirth. Writing in the spring of 1848,[48] he acknowledged that chloroform anaesthesia had an important place in surgery, 'few operations are now performed without it', and even claimed that within a fortnight of its introduction 'it was employed with due care by the most eminent surgeons in London'. But its use in midwifery was an entirely different matter. In order merely to relieve the natural pains of labour, 'patients are recklessly brought into a condition having between it and death the very narrowest limits'. Partly for this reason, the value of chloroform in midwifery had already 'declined in the estimation of those really able to judge'. Not everyone believed, like Simpson, that in all cases pain should be allayed, least of all 'pain attendant upon the natural process of parturition'. An eminent theologian, 'perhaps unequalled in learning', had explained that

> . . . the very infliction which touched the heart and imagination has been invested by Almighty God with a new and comfortable light, as being the medium of his choicest mercies towards us; pain . . . may be considered even as a blessing of the Gospel, and being a blessing, admits of being met well or ill.

This view coincided, it now appeared, with 'the conscientious convictions of parturient women'. Women were willing to suffer pain 'rather than act against their convictions'. There was no justification for compelling reluctant mothers to inhale chloroform when everyone knew that 'the most severe suffering for hours does not necessarily endanger life', and that 'since the time of Eve, the pains of labour have been endured by women'. Admittedly, mothers sometimes died in child-birth and prolonged pain must have something to do with this. But scientific midwifery will, sooner or later, 'effectually prevent the occurrence of death from the prolonged pains of labour'. Moreover, even the supporters of chloroform admit that its administration can produce 'ideas of a dreaming kind', and, said Gream,

> I do not hesitate to assert, that if women (Englishwomen) were put in possession, as they ought to be, of what [these ideas] consist in many instances, and what were the 'voluntary efforts made in accordance with them' that were made in more than once instance, before numerous witnesses, they would undergo even the most excruciating torture, or, I believe, suffer death itself, before they would subject themselves to the shadow of a chance of exhibitions such as have been recorded.

And Gream instanced the case of a patient of Dubois who (according to report) 'drew an attendant to her to kiss as she was in the second stage of narcotism'. Thus, and after all, the natural course of things is best; as it usually is. And for the truth of this doctrine Gream appealed to Denman, who had died 33 years before, but whose *Introduction to the Practice of Midwifery*, published in 1782, had gone into five editions and had been read, in their youth, by all the leading obstetricians of the late 1840s. According to Denman,

> in everything which relates to the act of parturition, Nature, not disturbed by disease, and unmolested by interruption, is fully competent to accomplish her own purpose; she may be truly said to disclaim and to abhor assistance . . . all women should believe, and find comfort in the reflection, that they are at those times under the peculiar care of Providence, and that their safety in child-birth is ensured by more numerous and powerful resources than under any other circumstances, though to appearance less dangerous.

This view, Gream went on, was well understood in London, and it was to the credit of his colleagues

> . . . that with but few exceptions anaesthesia has not been employed in midwifery in the metropolis — a circumstance tending to strengthen public confidence in London practitioners, and an assurance that by them human life is not recklessly hazarded. . . There are always those who, having nothing to lose, seek to gain reputation by

adopting novel practices and vague theories; but amongst others extensively engaged in practice, all that is not strictly legitimate is discarded; and this is the fate that the attempt to introduce anaesthesia in midwifery everywhere is meeting with.

A few paragraphs later, however, and the case is not so clear. 'I in no way recommend its hasty abolition in midwifery', because 'in some cases it may in time prove highly beneficial', especially if resort has to be had to instruments.

Like many others who took part in the debate, Gream was strong on indignation but short on facts. He alleged that chloroform retarded delivery; that it killed patients 'even when exhibited after the most approved principles'; that 'a feeling of aversion, to use no stronger term, pervades the minds of females of rank and education in this country, almost without exception, to the use of it'; once more the wretched guinea pig, killed twelve months before at the Royal Institution, was held out as an awful warning. On the other hand, he made the perhaps valid point that the advocates of chloroform tended to minimise its dangers while 'they designate as immoral the caution and judgment exercised by others less reckless than themselves'. Not being absolutely opposed to the use of chloroform, even in midwifery, he had kind words for John Snow, whose judicious and valuable observations, he said, were in marked contrast to the heedless claims and assertions of Professor Simpson.

There were in Gream traces of an open mind, containing some — although perhaps not very much — good judgment and common sense. A different kind of conservatism was shown by Meigs, Professor of Obstetrics at the Jefferson Medical College in Philadelphia. Meigs had graduated from the University of Pennsylvania in 1817, when Simpson was still a small boy, and by the 1840s was perhaps the most prominent obstetrician in America. Simpson wrote to Meigs concerning the use of chloroform in midwifery, and the substance of Meig's reply was published in the *Lancet* in June 1848.[49]

Meigs began by saying that in the United States chloroform was used in dentistry, and in surgery 'to a considerable extent', but that its use in midwifery 'has not as yet acquired a general vogue'. The Pennsylvania Hospital, with 200 beds, had never yet resorted to inhalation anaesthesia either in surgery or obstetrics. Meigs went on to explain that he likewise had never used chloroform or ether: 'I have not yielded to several solicitations as to its exhibition addressed to me by my patients in labour' and he gave three reasons for his decision. First, labour was a natural process:

> I have been accustomed to look upon the sensation of pain in labour
> as a physiological relative of the power or force . . . I have always
> regarded a labour-pain as a most desirable, salutary, and conservative
> manifestation of life-force. I have found that women, provided they
> were sustained by cheering counsel and promises, and carefully freed
> from the distressing element of terror, could in general be made to
> endure, without great complaint, those labour pains which the
> friends of anaesthesia desire so earnestly to abolish and nullify for
> all the fair daughters of Eve.

> There is no reasonable therapia of health. Hygienical processes are
> good and valid. The sick need a physician, not they that are well. To
> be in natural labour is the culminating point of the female somatic
> forces. There is, in natural labour, no element of disease — and there-
> fore the good old writers have said nothing truer nor wiser than their
> old saying, that 'a meddlesome midwifery is bad'.

Secondly, Meigs expressed a moral objection to the use of chloroform
on the ground that it produced a state undistinguishable from inebria-
tion:

> If I could believe that chloroformed insensibility is sleep indeed, the
> most considerable of my objections would vanish. Chloroform is not
> a soporific; and I see in the anaesthesia it superinduces a state of the
> nervous system in nowise differing from the anaesthetic results of
> alcoholic potations, save in the suddenness and transitiveness of its
> influence.

Thirdly, he believed — correctly — that chloroform was a dangerous
agent; but his explanation of the matter was wrapped up in arcane
physiology and honest rhetoric.

> . . . no law of succession of [the action of chloroform] on the
> several distinct parts of the brain has been or can hereafter ascer-
> tained. . .

> There are, indubitably, certain cases in which the intellectual hemi-
> spheres are totally hebetised and deprived of power by it, while the
> co-ordinating lobes remain perfectly unaffected. In others the motor-

cords of the cerebro-spinal nerves are deprived of power, while the sensitive cords enjoy a full activity, and *vice versa*.

Sometimes the influence of the agent upon the sources of the pneumogastric and phrenic nerves is dangerously, or at least alarmingly, made manifest by modification of the respiratory force . . . If continued but a little longer than the period required for hebitising the hemispheres, the cerebellum, the tubercula quadrigemina, and the cord, [the narcotising agent] overthrows the medulla oblongata, and thereby produces sudden death.

In these ominous-sounding circumstances Meigs felt that it was unjustifiable to use chloroform 'merely to prevent the physiological pain' and run the risk of killing the patient. Were he to lose a single patient in this way, Meigs wrote,

I should feel disposed to clothe me in sack-cloth, and cast ashes on my head for the remainder of my days. What sufficient motive have I to risk the life or the death of one in a thousand, in a questionable attempt to abrogate one of the general conditions of man?

These considerations applied to natural labour. As regards cases requiring the use of instruments Meigs relied on a different argument. This was not, as with some accoucheurs, that chloroform would increase an already serious danger of convulsions, but that the use of instruments would be far too difficult and dangerous if the patient could not tell what she felt:

No man can *absolutely* know the precise degree of inclination his patient will give to the plane of her superior strait while in pain — an inclination to be modified by every movement of her body and limbs. Under such absolute uncertainty, the best guide of the accoucheur is the reply of the patient to his interrogatory, 'Does it hurt you?' The patient's reply, 'Yes' and 'No', are worth a thousand dogmas and precepts as to planes and axes.

He refused, he said, to cast away, 'my safest and most trustworthy diagnosis'. Apparently it did not occur to him that a patient under chloroform, feeling no extreme pain, would not cause 'absolute uncertainty' through sudden spasmodic movements of body and limbs.

It has been said of Meigs that he was not an original thinker, and certainly his attitude to anaesthesia was entirely conservative. But it was not entirely unreasonable. It was true that there were risks in using chloroform, although they were very small if the anaesthetist knew what he was doing. It was true that no one understood just how chloroform worked. It was true that in the early nineteenth century a good obstetrician could make child-birth without anaesthesia bearable – could go a long way to preventing scenes of horror and desperation – by instilling confidence and cheerfulness into his patient as long as (and it is no small qualification) the labour was normal. Meigs was a very experienced obstetrician; he was kindly, careful and sympathetic, and he knew his work extremely well. To such a man, skilled in providing that moral support without which medical assistance is often of little use, chloroform was bound to seem, at best, a dubious step forward.

Gream and Meigs may be taken as fair representatives of the anti-anaesthesia-in-midwifery school. There were others whose statements were far more extreme. In 1850 Robert Barnes, lecturer in midwifery at the Hunterian School of Medicine and obstetric surgeon to the Western General Dispensary, entered the fray. Barnes was a man of commanding personality and considerable experience, and he had a good deal of influence. He was by no means convinced that chloroform should be used even in surgery. As to its use in midwifery, he considered that 'the agony of the pain occasioned by the stretching of the external parts' was beneficial 'because cries extorted from the mother by anguish too acute to bear in silence' took the strain off the perinaeum.[50] He also believed that exhibiting chloroform in midwifery caused convulsions, metritis, dysentry and other disorders. As late as 1853 Dr Robert Lee, lecturer in midwifery at St George's Hospital and a well-known writer on the subject, condemned as 'a most unnatural practice' the destruction of consciousness in women during labour, 'the pains and sorrows of which exerted a most powerful and salutary influence upon their religious and moral character, and upon all their future relations in life'. He further gave an account of seventeen cases that had come 'under his observation' in which chloroform ('this treacherous gift of science') had been used and had produced serious after-effects including peritonitis and 'insanity and great disturbance of the brain'. One of these patients had had difficulty in breathing for two weeks after delivery, and in another case Lee had been obliged to combat the residual chloroform in a patient's system for four months. Its use was, he said, 'an ignominious and disgraceful practice'. There had been 'systematic concealment of the truth . . . conceited or ignorant women of fashion made a pastime of this as of other quackeries . . . young and inexperienced mothers were decoyed to their destruction. . .'[51] This drew a sharp rejoinder even from John Snow. The expressions in the latter part of Dr Lee's paper, he said, 'were to be regretted'. And he added that Dr Lee's efforts at getting rid of the chloroform out of the system four months after it had been inhaled 'must have taken place at a time when the lady was no doubt quite as free from chloroform as Dr Lee himself'.[52]

Many and varied were the arguements brought forward. But even among medical men those most often heard were not about clinical experience but about the principles of proper behaviour; in particular, about God, Nature, and bad language. The last of these, admittedly, was a clinical experience of a kind. In 1848 Tyler Smith had found 'the occasional incitement of the sexual passion . . . under the influence of ether' a decidedly repulsive feature of anaesthesia.[53] In 1849 a speaker at the Westminster Medical Society referred to mothers using 'obscene and disgusting language'. This fact along he considered 'sufficient to prevent the use of chloroform in English women'.[54] (He also mentioned twelve cases of convulsion, five of mania, and 32 deaths all ascribable to chloroform.) Another report was of an operation 'on the vagina of a prostitute, in which [whom?] ether produced lascivious dreams'.[55] In the next few years there were several reports of 'scenes of an indelicate character', including the thought-provoking statement that 'delicate ladies will use language which it would be thought impossible they should ever have had an opportunity of hearing'.[56] Many doctors objected not so much to the bad language itself as to putting their patients into a situation in which they might use it, or, more often, they claimed that their patients would refuse to be put into such a situation. Others found abhorrent the idea that child-birth might be accompanied by sexual emotion. But less was heard of this kind of objection after the early 1850s.

What most obviously persisted was the feeling that painless childbirth was unnatural and improper, that pain was a natural and therefore a desirable concomitant of labour. On a simple logical level this argument was easy to deal with. Those who object to the use of chloroform in midwifery, Simpson wrote,

> wear clothes to assist the protecting influence of the skin, and do not think that 'unnatural'. They use cooking and condiments to aid the functions of mastication and digestion. . . They constantly ride in coaches etc as if the function of progression were imperfect in man. 'How unnatural', exclaimed an Irish lady to me lately, 'How

unnatural it is for you doctors in Edinburgh to take away the pains of your patients when in labour!' 'How unnatural', (said I) 'it is for you to have swimmed over from Ireland to Scotland against wind and tide in a steamboat!'[57]

The 'why interfere with a natural process?' argument was, up to a point, easy to deal with. If it held good for chloroform, then, as one writer to the *Lancet* put it, 'it would be wrong to interfere in midwifery at all — supporting the perinaeum, even, was not necessary, but meddle-some'.[58]

Answers of this kind, however, did not satisfy everyone. The analogy between travelling in a coach or a steamboat and giving birth to a child clearly leaves something to be desired; child-birth is, to say the least of it, a good deal more special. Thus it seemed to many people entirely reasonable to claim that God and Nature are intimately connected with parturition, and in a singular and sympathetic way. Nature, said Robert Barnes,

> . . . has secured the safety and the end of parturition through so many admirable provisions, that she may be truly said to disdain assistance, and to resent interference. . . It is an outrage upon the fundamental law of adaptation to assume that a beneficient Creator has associated pain with the parturient process for other than a wise and necessary purpose.[59]

Thus God and Nature walked hand in hand, and the 'anaesthetic or "meddling" school of midwifery' was — no one actually said this but it was clearly implied — an invention of the Devil. There was no denying that the pains of child-birth could be almost unbearable — 'it was clear enough that there were many women who would not flinch from surgical proceedings who expressed most bitterly the sufferings of parturition, which, though happening in the natural cause of things, were oftentimes all but intolerable, and were often made infinitely worse by being spread over so tedious a space'.[60] But the feeling that it was the duty of women, perhaps even their right, to suffer in this way ran very deep. In a sense, no doubt, this suffering elevated the sex; it gave to women an heroic quality which men could not match. If through chloroform they did not suffer, they were ordinary beings; child-birth was an ordinary event; chloroform reduced the status of woman, and changed the social order in a subtle but quite fundamental way. These ideas, if they were entertained, were entertained by men.

No woman spoke publicly on the subject, but there can be no doubt
that obstetricians were under pressure from their patients. One doctor
reported that a patient, 'after many hours of severe suffering', was
given chloroform and subsequently said, 'Up to the time of inhaling,
the pains were most severe, and were becoming insupportable; but they
appeared to do no good . . . I felt in despair . . .'[61] In such a situation,
no doctor would have found it easy to refuse relief, possibly helpful
relief. Meigs admitted[62] that 'several' patients in labour had asked for
chloroform, which he had refused. Barnes, one of the staunchest
opponents of anaesthesia in midwifery, reveals in the following passage,
evidently without being aware of it, that the contest was to some
extent between the mothers and the medical profession, as Simpson
had foretold:

> Women who were delivered before the discovery of anaesthetics
> have ceased to lament that they were born in an unhappy era. There
> is little apprehension, at least in this country, that the profession will
> be constrained, even against their better judgment, to employ nar-
> cotic vapour to satisfy the peremptory solicitations of their patients.
> The sense of professional responsibility here is too deep to allow of
> any such concession. The moral feeling of the women of England
> is too correct, and too elevated, to permit them to urge so im-
> proper a demand.[63]

This could not have been written if there had been no 'peremptory
solicitations' from patients. We know from case histories that there
were mothers, even in England, who were only too glad to inhale
chloroform. And Barnes's appeal to the correctness and elevation of
the moral feelings of the women of England is, to some extent at least,
an appeal to imaginary evidence to support his own opinions and prejudices.

While these arguments went on, chloroform continued to be used,
and medical evidence accumulated to prove that, besides allaying pain,
chloroform properly administered made labour easier and shorter,
and therefore safer, and that it had no unfavourable after-effects.
Understanding gradually spread that it was of little use to talk about
administering or not administering chloroform; what mattered was
how much was administered and how it was administered. As early as
the summer of 1848, this was clearly recognised by others besides
Simpson and Snow. Dr E.W. Murphy observed that chloroform 'does
not interfere with the action of the uterus, unless given in very large

doses, which is never necessary'. Properly used, 'it causes a greater relaxation in the passages and perinaeum; the mucous secretion from the vagina is also increased. It subdues the nervous irritation caused by severe pain, and restores nervous energy. It secures the patient perfect repose for some hours after her delivery'.[64] Eighteen months later Murphy repeated these points, giving the results in 21 cases using chloroform:

> The uterus was not paralysed in a single case; in one case the period between the pains was lengthened, but the action of the uterus was more efficient; in another case the labour appeared to be retarded and the uterine contractions came on more quickly and forcibly when the chloroform was omitted, but in all cases its contractile power was by no means lessened. The 78 cases recorded by Dr Channing proved the same.[65]

Reports of the beneficial effects of chloroform, especially in difficult or retarded delivery, accumulated. Many opponents remained unconvinced; but they could not produce countervailing evidence. Above all, it was increasingly clear that chloroform could hardly be refused to mothers on grounds of safety. 'It should be remembered', John Snow was reported as saying in 1853,

> . . . that no death from chloroform had occurred in midwifery, and he knew of only one case where the patient was in danger, and that arose from gross mismanagement, for the husband was giving the chloroform, and looking another way.[66]

Technical backwardness or a dubious morality; these were what seemed the foundations of anti-anaesthesia by the middle of the 1850s, and on these foundations it could not survive. Seven or eight years of experience of anaesthesia were enough. As Simpson had prophesied near the beginning, it was the facts that were decisive.

This long debate about chloroform — it was almost over by the middle of the 1850s — was a rambling and confused affair. It would have lasted longer, and it would have been even more confused, had it not been dominated by Simpson and Snow. From the very first Simpson was resolved to triumph. He believed in the cause and he believed in the drug. If he had never lived and chloroform anaesthesia had not been discovered (no doubt it would have been discovered, but later than 1847) ether would in due course have spread into general surgical and obstetric use in Great Britain. But its spread, without the powerful influence of a strong and eager controversialist like Simpson to support it, would probably have been slower than was the spread of chloroform. No doubt Simpson's domineering style was counter-productive in some quarters. But deep conviction, allied to his considerable practical experience, his crusading zeal, his prestige as a professor in a famous medical school, and not least to the desperate need of patients, enabled Simpson to bear down the opposition. Moreover, what Simpson lacked in finesse and scientific skill was made up for by the brilliance, modesty and perseverance of John Snow. Snow was completely confident in using ether in 1847,[67] and early in 1848 he went on record as saying that chloroform was superior to ether as an anaesthetic. Its use, he said in 1849, 'was attended with no risk whatever' in skilled hands. Opponents of chloroform who brushed Simpson's arguments aside seldom if ever failed to listen to Snow. Syme's influence was probably also considerable, even in London. In February 1849, he told the Medico-Chirurgical Society of Edinburgh that he

 . . . strongly advocated the use of chloroform in surgery generally. After it was proposed by Dr Simpson, he used it in the first operation he had to perform in the hospital, and ever since then he had continued the practice. Further, he desired at this time to state to the Society, that he believed anaesthesia not only saved patients operated on from pain, but also from shock, and all its effects. When Dr Simpson first stated this as his opinion, he (Mr Syme) strongly opposed it; but now he was convinced that Dr Simpson was right in his opinion.[68]

Chloroform, Syme said, was 'constantly employed' in Edinburgh both in surgery and obstetrics and there had been no fatality. Syme had a way in his lectures of combining experience with reasonableness that was very persuasive. It was perhaps unfortunate that he added (perhaps with the London debates in mind, and perhaps not without malice) that he was inclined to think that the accounts of sexual excitement under chloroform were 'the result of impressions harboured in the minds of the practitioners, not in the minds of the chloroformed'.[69]

For a controversy that depended, or should have depended, to a large degree on facts, two features stand out. The first is the near-absence of statistics and the total absence of worth-while statistics. Simpson produced some figures in December 1847, in support of his view that it was 'fundamentally unsound' to say that pain was useful.

The figures relate to the Dublin Maternity Hospital, and are as follows:[70]

    1 mother in 320 died when labour terminated within 2 hours
    1 mother in 145 died when labour terminated within 2–6 hours
    1 mother in 80 died when labour terminated within 7–12 hours
    1 mother in 26 died when labour terminated within 12–24 hours
    1 mother in 17 died when labour terminated within 24–36 hours
    1 mother in 6 died when labour terminated in over 36 hours

He also produced figures for amputations of the thigh in various hospitals in Great Britain, Ireland and France which were to the effect that:

| | | | |
|---|---|---|---|
| 'in the hospitals of Paris', | 1836–41, | 201 cases, | 63 in 100 died |
| in Edinburgh | 1839–42, | 43 cases, | 49 in 100 died |
| cases reported by Phillips, | 1844, | 435 cases, | 44 in 100 died |
| cases reported by Lawrie (Glasgow), | | 127 cases, | 36 in 100 died |

whereas he himself had notes of 145 cases using ether in which the death rate was 25 in 100.[71] Robert Barnes replied to this and correctly pointed out that 'the statistical professor' proved nothing with his statistics about the effects and duration of labour or about mortality in amputations of the thigh simply because there were so many other variables involved of which Simpson took no account whatever. In 1848 Barnes, who seems himself to have had some interest in statistics, remarked that claims that chloroform diminished mortality in childbirth were 'premature, if not absurd', and that at least 10,000 cases would have to be recorded before such a deduction could be drawn. In 1855 Dr James Arnott, who was unenthusiastic about chloroform because he was trying to popularise local refrigeration of the part, produced a table, said to have been printed in the *American Journal of the Medical Sciences* in April 1852, giving the following figures for 'New York, Boston and Philadelphia':

### Death Rates in Amputations

| *Wounds* | | *Chronic Diseases* | |
|---|---|---|---|
| with anaesthetics, | 1 in 3.4 | with anaesthetics, | 1 in 6.7 |
| without anaesthetics, | 1 in 2.2 | without anaesthetics, | 1 in 5 |

This is rather surprising, because Simpson was certainly fond of what he called 'the evidence of statistical observation'. But, like almost everyone else who used statistics at all, he used them in a very cavalier fashion. Thus in a controversy which raged in 1847, Simpson, in order to prove that turning the child during labour was highly dangerous, quoted figures for cases reported by West (17 cases), Churchill (174 cases), and another fourteen authors reporting a total of 654 cases. These authors included Paul Portal, whose *La Pratique des Accoucheurs* was published in 1685. He also relied on the fact that Robert Lee, in his *Midwifery Lectures*, published in 1844, reported 72 cases from four different sources. This readiness to quote figures from several countries and several centuries, as if they were all equally reliable, and also to quote the figures of A as reported by B, is remarkable enough. But also, as Lee pointed out, a case of placental presentation might be of several kinds and include a variety of other complications, and the mortality figures which Simpson quoted could therefore not be taken as indicating the dangers of placental presentation as such. Careless reporting and careless use of statistics was the rule. In 1849 Simpson was accused by Robert Collins, Master of the Lying-in Hospital in Dublin, of saying that the death rate in the Edinburgh Maternity Hospital for 1844–6 was 1 in 134 (1 in 368 excluding puerperal fever) whereas the Report of the Hospital gave the figure as 1 in 53.5. In reply, Simpson pointed out that his figure was for all the deliveries 'under the superintendence of the institution' whereas 1 in 53.5 referred to in-patients only. Simpson also observed that in comparing mortalities allowance had to be made for the occurrence of epidemic deaths from puerperal fever. Collins, he said, had referred to 'Professor Hamilton's frightful mortality' of 1 in 21. But in 1821–2 'puerperal fever raged extensively in Edinburgh . . . it is to this period of misfortune that Dr Collins's ungenerous remark on the fatality of Dr Hamilton's practice refers' – and even so, Collins has stated 1 in 21 when it was 1 in 30. What Collins actually stated was 1 in 22.

The second feature of the chloroform controversy that must strike a modern reader with astonishment is its tone. From first to last it throve on emotion and inaccuracy. Concerning anaesthesia in surgery there was little argument and perhaps even less emotion. But writing about etherisation in midwifery in 1847 Simpson was already castigating opponents for conservatism, inhumanity and unscrupulous misuse of evidence, and implying that they were ready to 'traffic in the perpetuation of human sufferings'. Some of his followers admired him for anticipating opposition, but his way of meeting it probably did no good. It was true, of course, that the medical profession as a whole was conservative and old-fashioned, and Simpson was not the only one to say so. Syme's lectures published in 1855 contain the following comment:

This operation [external incision of the urethra] when first proposed, met with violent opposition, but this is no more than was to be expected; for a new proposal of any value is sure to be strongly opposed, while useless and injurious ones are, curiously enough, often received with great favour. . . I may remind you of the strong opposition made to Harvey's theory of the circulation of the blood, and again to vaccination . . . five and twenty years ago excision of the elbow-joint had not yet been performed in Great Britain, and when I first adopted it the most vehement opposition was raised. The late Mr Liston, in this theatre, characterised it as a blackguard operation, but it has since come to be generally adopted.[72]

Medical conservatism also showed itself in a readiness to appeal to authority, ancient or modern. Gream's appeal to the authority of Denman has already been quoted. Late in 1849 one of the strongest objections urged against the use of chloroform in midwifery was that 'Collins, Meigs, Montgomery and others' were against it. This sometimes combined with an astonishing capacity to be satisfied with evidence from long ago. In the placental presentation controversy one writer described at length a caesarian operation carried out by John Hunter in 1774 ('about the time when he was publishing his plates of the gravid uterus') and, at even greater length, a similar operation carried out early in the nineteenth century by John Bell and written up by Sir Charles Bell in *Medico-Chirurgical Transactions* in 1813.[73] This was in 1847. The writer made no reference to any observations of his own.[74]

This was not unusual. Those who argued against chloroform in midwifery but had never tried it were fond of quoting, and sometimes enlarging upon, the disastrous experiences of their colleagues who had. In 1849 a Dr Webster, who 'had no personal experience' of chloroform in either surgery or midwifery, reported three cases which had 'come within his cognisance'. In each of these there had been subsequent ill-effects, one patient becoming 'perfectly maniacal, and so furious, as to require confinement in a lunatic asylum, where she remained for twelve months, when she was discharged cured'.[75] No evidence was provided to show that the mania was the result of the chloroform, and the speaker did not know the details of the case. Another doctor — this time, surprisingly, from Scotland — who had never used chloroform but was impressed by Wakley's experiments, referred to the 'fearful risk' and 'unseemly scenes' caused by using chloroform in child-birth, the 'numerous mishaps' and 'fatal cases . . . wonderfully smoothed by a ready pen'.[76] No instances or figures were given. Barnes's 1850 onslaught on the use of chloroform was based on 27 cases reported by Dr Sachs in the Berlin Lying-in Hospital.

A conservative profession facing one of the greatest changes in practice ever proposed, and unaccustomed to sifting and weighing evidence was bound to be alarmed and confused. Many of its leaders became excited, and rudeness and rhetoric often took the place of reason and observation. 'Has chloroform not yet had its full allotment of victims?' wrote one doctor in 1848. 'Is the anaesthetic mania not yet over?'[77] 'Surely', wrote another, 'Dr Barnes can teach his pupils much more certain means of making out [a] diagnosis by the use of their fingers, than by insisting upon the patients continuing to shriek in order that he and his pupils may take it out by the use of their ears?'[78] Barnes, in his turn, rejected Simpson's assurance that chloroform was safe because he had used it on himself; the professor at that time, he said, 'was not in labour'. A few years later, when the opponents of chloroform were beginning to lose ground, Snow tried to explain to Robert Lee just what chloroform could and could not do, and just how much should be exhibited for different purposes; the answer was that sniffing 15 drops on a handkerchief ('the way chloroform was administered by Dr Snow in natural labour') was 'a mere pretence, and calculated only to deceive the weak, ignorant and credulous'.[79] This was 'chloroform *à la reine'* humbug. He, Dr Lee, was talking about 'real anaesthesia', which was nothing more nor less than a futile attempt to abrogate an ordinance of the Almighty, 'In sorrow shalt thou bring forth children'.[80]

The proponents of chloroform were not behindhand in the exchange of insults. Simpson had a particularly impressive command of language, and this was in evidence even before the discovery of chloroform. In the placental presentation controversy of 1847 he wrote:

> It is a well-known fact, that when the cuttle-fish wishes to escape and hide itself, it empties its sepia or ink-bag, so as to darken the surrounding water, and cover its retreat. In his last paper Dr Lee has scattered his ink upon the pages of the *Lancet* with apparently a similar object.[81]

He then replied to Lee's paper point by point — 'into these consecutive sentences Dr Lee has managed, with his usual ingenuity, to compress five separate and distinct errors of statement' — in a way which leaves a modern reader almost totally at a loss to know whether Lee was or was not as great a fool as Simpson made him out to be. There is a swashbuckling rhetorical grandeur in Simpson's style of argument that is both overwhelming and impressive. He never let a point go. His reading and resource were enormous, and everything was said that could be said to make his adversaries look small and their lives disagreeable.

These talents Simpson employed with great skill, but not necessarily with the best effect, in the chloroform controversy. Because he tended to treat opponents as if they were either knavish or stupid, many reasonable men reacted against his views. To Simpson, chloroform was a revelation; and for those who were ready to believe there was no difficulty. Dr Simpson's arguments, one doctor wrote in 1848, 'are unanswerable, and put the matter beyond a doubt'.[82] Such views were to be found usually, although not always, in Scotland; and for this there was a reason. Simpson was a Scotsman, working in Edinburgh, and to the Scots it was important that he was one of themselves. But to many Englishmen he was a pushing, noisy, innovative, combative member of a medical school which was often regarded, especially in London, as upstart and eccentric. Simpson was certainly quite right in saying in 1847 (and it showed great prescience) that many medical men would feel that 'established medical opinions and medical practices should not be harshly interfered with'. But at least some of the opposition was to himself. Gream's 1848 assault on the use of chloroform in midwifery — a 2,500-word article — was at most one-third argument and approximately one-third protest against Simpson's campaign and, more generally, against his life style and way of doing things. Does it show a healthy state of the profession, Gream asked, when discoveries in medicine are made the medium for general agitating purposes? Is it right that the ordinary journals of daily news should be the sources through which information of medical improvements is given to the profession? Was the use of the stethoscope, or the discovery of Bright's disease of the kidney, first made known through the columns of the *Morning Post*? Not content with criticising Simpson's methods of persuasion, Gream went on to imply that financial embarrassment was the real reason for Simpson's activity:

> . . . the constant desire for publicity, as the performer of some new operation, the deliverer of women by some novel process, and the author of extravagant and totally inapplicable remedies for uterine diseases — the repetition of pamphlets, correspondence with newspapers, and the absences from home, sometimes to attend exclusively single cases of midwifery, at others to exhibit the wonderful effects of chloroform for the amusement of individuals [give] the impression of a narrowed rather than an extended practice.[83]

This libellous suggestion was totally and absolutely untrue, as Gream was very swiftly informed; 'Professor Simpson has not been able to overtake all the practice which flows in upon him', wrote James Moffat. But Gream went on to lecture the discoverer of chloroform anaesthesia as if he were addressing an apothecary's apprentice in a parish poorhouse:

> Let those who think to rise by agitation 'take heed they fall' . . . [Denman, Osborn and Clarke] — their names have never appeared in advertisements as patronising the inventions of stay-makers, nor have they permitted them to form the prominent features of druggists' announcements; their conduct has never tended to convert their profession into a trade. . .

Gream's complaint was now quite clear. Simpson was an outsider, he didn't know how to behave. It is not an accident that the word 'propriety' was so often used, in several connections, by many of those who took part in the chloroform controversy.

As to the spreading use of anaesthesia, this cannot be traced with precision. Early in 1847 ether was being used successfully in many operations throughout the country, and the same can be said of chloroform from early in 1848. Progress in England was slower than in Scotland. One reason seems to have been that English chloroform was less pure than that made in Edinburgh where, from the beginning, the local supplier, Duncan and Flockhart, had most of the market and was in close touch with the university. This was not the situation elsewhere, and according to the *Scotsman* demand for chloroform in the last few months of 1847 was so great that 'in Edinburgh, London, Liverpool and other towns many [chemists] have been up all night distilling it'; such efforts, doubtless by the skilled, the semi-skilled, and the almost unskilled, can hardly have failed to produce many gallons of inferior or even dangerous liquid. Another reason for slower progress in England seems to have been that English surgeons, having less conviction about chloroform anaesthesia than the Scots, administered chloroform in smaller doses, and more gradually, and then stopped at an early stage, mistaking the strugglings of the half-anaesthetised patient for 'delirium, spasms, convulsions, and failure'. But by the spring of 1848 even Gream, no doubt referring to London, admitted that 'few operations are now performed without it'.[84] Also in 1848 *Punch* carried the story of 'a medical man, of the very old school, who calls all operations that are performed without the patient feeling anything, "senseless operations" '.[85] This does not sound as if 'the very old school' was by then more than a remnant. The report of a fatality under chloroform at Manchester in 1853 begins with the words, 'Almost every patient takes it'.[86] In some quarters, the view persisted for several years that chloroform should be used only in severe operations, but this became more and more a minority opinion. Experience of its use in the Crimean war virtually ended opposition among surgeons, a good deal after it was realised that chloroform not only made operations safer but also brought within reach of the surgeon a whole array of operations 'which, without the assistance of this agent, could not be thought of'.[87]

It was a different matter in midwifery. Simpson used ether early in 1847 and Protheroe Smith used ether in England only a few weeks later. Simpson used chloroform in midwifery as soon as he had discovered the possibility, and it was being used at the Bristol General Hospital very early in 1848. By the end of 1848 chloroform was used in midwifery in London to a modest extent, and in 1849 there are references in the *Lancet* to scores of cases, no doubt indicating its use in hundreds more. But 'a very strong prejudice in England against chloroform in midwifery' was reported.[88] This was due in part to the caution and conservatism shown by leading English obstetricians, but also to the fact that in England the apothecaries played a far larger role than in Scotland —

> men destitute of a liberal education — the majority of them having no education at all beyond a provincial school until they went to walk the hospitals — and their system of practice is to pander to the prejudices and to flatter the ignorance of their drug-swallowing patients.[89]

In 1850 Robert Barnes declared that doubts about safety were growing, but there is little evidence of this; after all, the fatalities attributed to chloroform that continued to occur were not in child-birth. What did keep growing was the evidence of successful use, and the number of unemotional communications recording this. For example, in 1853 W. Martin Coates, Surgeon to the Salisbury Infirmary, wrote to say that chloroform was a dangerous agent but was perfectly safe if administered 'in the smallest possible quantity consistent with success'. He used it, he said, in natural labour 'when the patient desires it, and circumstances do not forbid it. In operative midwifery, I recommend it.[90] Calm, assured, practical, unrhetorical, Martin Coates's statement, and others like it, avoided the gladiatorial element in the discussions and must have seemed to many to be persuasive common sense.

Physicians who did not feel perfect confidence in the agent — it is almost certain that there were not many of these in Scotland — or who were against moderating the pains of child-birth as a matter of principle, could adopt the position first indicated in 1848, that chloroform need not be used if the patient 'did not suffer greatly from the expulsive efforts; if she did not complain of the pains being more than she could bear; if the process of labour promised to be of short duration'.[91] In other words, there were doctors who did not use chloroform in normal labour if it could be avoided. This may have been a common attitude in 1848, but it is doubtful if it was still widespread among thoughtful physicians in 1853. It was therefore the residual opponents of chloroform in midwifery who learned with dismay that on 8 April 1853, Queen Victoria had given birth to a son and that chloroform had been administered by John Snow. The use of chloroform may have been the Queen's decision or it may have been Prince Albert's. In any case, it set an example which every woman in the country felt she had a right to follow, for Prince Albert would never have agreed to it if he had thought it dangerous, and the Queen would never have agreed to it if she had thought it against the will of God. As for the doctors, many must have known that Her Majesty's physician, Sir James Clark, was not likely to have urged anything as modern as the use of chloroform on a reluctant Queen. Clark, who had been a naval surgeon after qualifying at Edinburgh, was an enthusiast for the restorative powers of fresh air, and practised Gregorian physic — free blood letting, brisk purging, frequent blisters, and vomits of tartar emetic. A few years earlier, in 1839, he had been generally (although perhaps wrongly) convicted of serious incompetence in suggesting that one of the Queen's ladies-in-waiting, Lady Flora Hastings, was pregnant when in fact, as time all too soon showed, she was dying of a liver tumour. (Subsequently, he was to be accused of mishandling the typhoid that killed Prince Albert.) Sir James, notably discreet and immensely influential, was not an advanced thinker: he published some books but made, it has been said, 'no addition to medical knowledge'; but even if the chloroform decision was taken by others, he had at least known enough to call in John Snow. The Queen made no secret of the fact that she had found Dr Snow's services of great value — she knew what she was talking about, for this was her eighth confinement — and Simpson, to whom Clark wrote giving the news, was jubilant. Three years before, when Prince Arthur had been born, chloroform had not been used.

The daily newspapers along with the *Associated Medical Journal* (later the *British Medical Journal*) emphasised the fact that chloroform had been administered. There were those to whom the news was unwelcome. In the official list of doctors attending the Queen, Snow's name was not included and the *Lancet* (still edited by Wakley who had drawn up the etherisation questionnaire in 1847) actually denied that chloroform had been used. Its editorial on the subject is interesting.

A very extraordinary report has obtained general circulation. . . Intense astonishment has been excited throughout the profession by the rumour that her Majesty during her last labour was placed under the influence of chloroform, an agent which has unquestionably caused instantaneous death in a considerable number of cases . . . we could not imagine that anyone had incurred the awful responsibility of ordering the administration of chloroform to her Majesty during a perfectly natural labour with a seventh [should read eighth] child. On inquiry, therefore, we were not at all surprised to learn that in her late confinement the Queen was not rendered insensible by chloroform or by any other anaesthetic agent. We state this with feelings of the highest satisfaction. In no case could it be justifiable to administer chloroform in perfectly ordinary labour. . . Probably some officious meddler about the Court so far overruled her Majesty's responsible professional advisers as to lead to the pretence of administering chloroform. . . Let it not be supposed that we would under-value the immense importance of chloroform in surgical operations . . . but inasmuch as it has destroyed life in a considerable number of instances, its *unnecessary* inhalation involves, in our opinion, an amount of responsibility which words cannot adequately describe.

We have felt irresistibly impelled to make the foregoing observations, fearing the consequences of allowing such a rumour respecting a dangerous practice in one of our national palaces to pass unrefuted. Royal examples are followed with extraordinary readiness by a certain class of society in this country.

Alas for the *Lancet's* peace of mind, everyone soon knew that this 'extraordinary report' was true. Snow and Simpson and chloroform in natural labour had triumphed. What the Queen did in this matter must have had some effect on the ultra-conservative doctors in London who practised in the upper reaches of society. It probably made little difference in Birmingham or Bethnal Green, no difference in Scotland. And a few remained unpersuaded, even by royal example. In 1856, the

*Lancet* printed 48 lectures by Tyler Smith on the 'Theory and Practice of Obstetrics'. There are only two references to chloroform. One refers to the fact that chloroform, like opium and emetic tartar, has 'relaxing effects'.[92] The other is an incidental reference to 'accoucheurs who approve the use of chloroform in labour'.[93] But the game was up. After years of dispute, of appeal to every defensible and to several indefensible principles on earth and — allegedly — in the heavens above, chloroform anaesthesia had become, as far as practicable, every mother's right, and every doctor's duty.

## Notes

1. J.C. Warren, *Effects of Chloroform and of Strong Chloric Ether* (Boston, 1849), p. 5.

2. *Lancet*, vol. I, (1848), pp. 19—21.

3. Ibid., p. 179.

4. *London Medical Gazette*, vol. XII, (1851), p. 626.

5. B.W. Richardson, in John Snow, *On Chloroform and Other Anaesthetics*, (ed. Richardson) (London, 1858), p. xvii.

6. *Lancet*, vol. I, (1847), p. 321.

7. *London Medical Gazette*, vol. VI, (1848), p. 255.

8. *Lancet*, vol. II, (1848), p. 46.

9. *Lancet* vol. I, (1854), p. 534.

10. *Lancet*, vol. I, (1853), p. 523.

11. *Lancet*, vol. I, (1848), p. 163.

12. *Lancet*, vol. I, (1855), p. 55.

13. *Lancet*, vol. I, (1848), p. 175.

14. Ibid., p. 179.

15. *London Medical Gazette*, vol. VI, (1848), p. 277.

16. *Lancet*, vol. I, (1855), p. 55.

17. *Lancet*, vol. II, (1847), p. 550.

18. J.Y. Simpson, *Anaesthesia, Hospitalism and other Papers* (ed. W.G. Simpson) (Edinburgh), p. 179.

19. *Lancet*, vol. I, (1855), p. 56.

20. *Lancet*, vol. I, (1848), p. 48.

21. *Lancet*, vol. I, (1855), p. 591.

22. Snow, *On Chloroform and other Anaesthetics*, p. 79.

23. *Lancet*, vol. I, (1855), p. 108.

24. F. Magendie, quoted in M. Duncum, *Development of Inhalation Anaesthesia* (Oxford, 1947), p. 159.

25. *Lancet*, vol. II, (1855), p. 367.

26. *Lancet*, vol II, (1872), p. 404.

27. *Lancet*, vol. I, (1851), p. 54.

28. Quoted in J.Y. Simpson, *Remarks on the Superinduction of Anaesthesia in Natural and Morbid Parturition* (Edinburgh, 1847), pp. 7—8.

29. *Lancet*, vol. I, (1848), p. 123.

30. Ibid., p. 205, letter from Dr J. Henry Bennet.

31. *Lancet*, vol. II, (1847), p. 549.

32. *Scotsman*, 27 November 1847.

33. 'Notes on the Employment of the Inhalation of Sulphuric Ether in the Practice of Midwifery', in *Monthly Journal of Medical Science*, no. 75 (March, 1847), pp. 721 ff.

34. *Lancet*, vol. I, (1847), pp. 321–3.

35. *Lancet*, vol. II, (1847), p. 452. Inducing premature labour was pioneered in Britain by John Denman in the 1770s and 1780s. It was therefore not sanctified by very long usage.

36. J.Y. Simpson, *Remarks on the Superinduction of Anaesthesia* (Edinburgh, 1848), p. 5.

37. J.Y. Simpson, *Account of a New Anaesthetic Agent* (Edinburgh, 1847), p. 14.

38. 'Cases of the Employment of Chloroform in Midwifery; with Remarks', in *Lancet*, vol. II, (1847), p. 623.

39. Ibid., p. 677.

40. J.Y. Simpson, *Answer to the Religious Objections Advanced Against the Employment of Anaesthetic Agents in Midwifery and Surgery* (Edinburgh, 1848), p. 13.

41. Draft letter to Protheroe Smith, undated, probably 1848.

42. Draft letter to Protheroe Smith.

43. *Lancet*, vol. II, (1848), p. 128.

44. *Lancet*, vol. I, (1848), p. 229.

45. Ibid., p. 443.

46. Ibid., p. 254.

47. Ibid., p. 477.

48. *Lancet*, vol. I, (1849), pp. 228 ff. Also G.T. Gream, *Remarks on the Employment of Anaesthetic Agents in Midwifery* (London, 1848).

49. *Lancet*, vol. I, (1848), pp. 613–4.

50. *Lancet*, vol. II, (1850), p. 39.

51. *Lancet*, vol. II, (1853), p. 608.

52. Ibid.,

53. *Supra*, p. 97.

54. *Lancet*, vol. I, (1849), p. 100.

55. Ibid.

56. *Lancet*, vol. I, (1856), p. 424.

57. Draft letter to Protheroe Smith, 1848.

58. *Lancet*, vol. I, (1848), p. 477.

59. R. Barnes in *Lancet*, vol. II, (1850), p. 39.

60. *Lancet*, vol. II, (1849), p. 537.

61. *Lancet*, vol. II, (1848), p. 182.

62. *Supra*, p. 106.

63. *Lancet*, vol. II (1850), p. 82.

64. *Lancet*, vol. I, (1848), p. 392.

65. *Lancet*, vol. II, (1849), p. 508.

66. Ibid., p. 537.

67. See *On the Inhalation of the Vapour of Ether in Surgical Operations . . . and a Statement of the Results of nearly Eighty Operations in which Ether has been Employed* (London, 1847).

68. Reported in *Lancet*, vol. I, (1849), p. 235.

69. This seems to have been the Edinburgh view. Simpson once observed that the obscene language argument 'has been repeated and gloated over by those who have propounded it, in a way forming, apparently unconsciously on their part, the severest self-inflicted censure upon the sensuality of their own thoughts'. *Anaesthetic Midwifery: Report on its Early History and Progress* (Edinburgh, 1848), p. 19.

70. *Lancet*, vol. II, (1848), p. 537.
71. See *Lancet*, vol. II, (1847), p. 625.
72. *Lancet*, vol. I, (1855), p. 28.
73. *Medico-Churgical Transactions, Medical and Chirurgical Society of London*, vol. IV, 1813, pp. 347–51.
74. *Lancet*, vol. II, (1847), p. 250.
75. *Lancet*, vol. II, (1849), p. 538.
76. *Lancet*, vol. II, (1848), p. 181.
77. Ibid.
78. *Lancet*, vol. I, (1848), p. 97.
79. Snow was content to exhibit chloroform on a handkerchief in natural labour, because all that he aimed for was a diminution of common sensibility, not 'complete anaesthesia'.
80. *Lancet*, vol. II, (1853), p. 609.
81. *Lancet*, vol. II, (1847), p. 517.
82. *Lancet*, vol. I, (1848), p. 240.
83. Ibid., p. 229.
84. Ibid., p. 228.
85. *Lancet*, vol. II, (1854), p. 513.
86. *Lancet*, vol. I, (1853), p. 21.
87. *Lancet*, vol. I, (1852), p. 329.
88. Letter from Dr A.W. Cockburn to Simpson, 30 January 1849; in the Library of the Royal College of Surgeons, Edinburgh.
89. Letter from Dr Cockburn to Simpson, ibid.
90. *Lancet*, vol. I, (1853), pp. 491–2.
91. *Lancet*, vol. I, (1848), p. 476.
92. *Lancet*, vol. II, (1856), p. 240.
93. Ibid., p. 646.

# 4 GERMS, INFLAMMATION AND ANTISEPSIS

In his *Herball or Generall Historie of Plants* published in 1597, Gerard describes the generation of the barnacle goose. He relates how — as had been believed for several hundred years — the barnacle goose breeds not from an egg, like other birds, but from a shell-fish, namely the ship's barnacle. These shell-fish, he explains, grow like fruit on the branches of certain trees standing by the edge of the sea. As the fruit ripen, the little goslings emerge, which, if they fall into the sea, swim away, but unfortunately die if they fall on land. The book contains a picture of this goose-tree with five great tulip-like barnacles attached, and several little goslings swimming about in the water below. The tree, Gerard tells his readers, grows in remote places such as the small Isle of Fouldrey in Morecombe Bay, and he describes it exactly, not as some traveller's tale, doubtfully recalled, but as something he had seen himself.

This kind of belief about the origins of living things amounted to a denial of the fundamental general principle of modern biology that all organisms, certainly all higher organisms, are self-reproducing. Earlier ages, on the contrary, believed that while this was quite obviously true in general, it was a rule that admitted a variety of exceptions. The barnacle goose was one. Another occurred when one sort of organism gave birth to creatures of a quite different kind. Even human beings, it was thought, might be subject to this sort of lapse or heterodoxy of nature. Thus when a woman in London, early in the eighteenth century, announced that she had given birth to rabbits, a large number of people, including some doctors, believed her. Such a story, one hundred years later, would have been met with general incredulity. But there continued into the days of Queen Victoria, even in the best-educated circles, the conviction that some kinds of creatures could be generated spontaneously within decaying matter. This belief went back at least to classical times.

In the second half of the seventeenth century knowledge increased, and the foundations of micro-biology began to be laid. An Italian physician, Francesco Redi, showed in a series of convincing experiments that maggots do not appear spontaneously in decaying flesh but come from eggs laid there by flies. This result was of limited value, however, because it was not generalised — on the contrary, Redi maintained that the grubs in oak galls, for example, were a case of spontaneous genera-

127

tion. Almost at the same time, a very significant scientific discovery was made in Holland. Van Leeuwenhoek, a draper by trade, ground lenses in his spare time and mounted them in his own microscopes. In 1676 he described, in one of a long series of letters to the Royal Society in London, how he had observed through a microscope four different kinds of minute living creatures in rain water:

> The fourth sort of animalcules which I saw moving about were so small that, for all of me, no shape can be specified. These animalcules were more than a thousand times smaller than the eye of a full-grown louse. . . They exceed in speed the previously described animalcules. I have at various times seen them stopping at one point, and whirling themselves at a speed such as we see in a spinning top before our eye; and then again motion in a circle, the circumference of which was hardly greater than that of a small sand-grain; and then again either straight out or in a crooked path.[1]

These were possibly protozoa. Some years later, however, van Leeuvenhoek described minute organisms which were undoubtedly bacteria, probably obtained from his own mouth. Some appeared motionless, but others had 'a very strong and swift motion, and shot through the liquid like a pike does through water'. Thus for the first time the marvellous world of microbes was seen by man.

This was in a sense a great discovery. But as with many discoveries its practical importance was at the time in no way realised. Neither van Leeuwenhoek nor any of his contemporaries surmised that knowledge of these tiny animalcules might be useful in combating disease; indeed, there was not in his own writing even the least suggestion that what he had observed might be related to the causes of human illness. Early in the eighteenth century the possibility of such a connection was glimpsed. A Dr Benjamin Marten, 'an obscure practitioner who lived in Theobald's Row', observed in 1720 that there might exist 'wonderfully minute living creatures that, by their peculiar Shape or disagreeable Parts are inimicable to our Nature, but, however, capable of subsisting in our Juices and Vessels';[2] but few doctors showed any interest. Even Linnaeus, who was a physician, in the 1767 edition of his *Systema Naturae* placed van Leeuwenhoek's animalcules in a class which he designated 'Chaos', grouping them along with 'the ethereal clouds suspended in the sky in the month of blossoming'.[3]

Working without any knowledge of the significance of bacteria, it was impossible for physicians to obtain much understanding of the onset and spread of disease. Opinion on this subject in the eighteenth century was essentially not much different from what had been taught by Hippocrates and Galen. According to these writers, the principal cause of illness is bad air containing poisonous miasmas derived from evil-smelling swamps and decaying animal matter. Neither Galen nor Hippocrates made clear the precise nature of the noxious exhalations, and there was no explanation of the fact, which was recognised in an off-hand way, that many diseases seemed to be communicable. But during the Middle Ages increasing attention was paid to the problem of communication. Giovanni Boccaccio, in the *Decameron,* described the terrible Florentine plague of 1348 and referred to the disease as a contagion:

> not only did converse and consorting with the sick give to the sound infection or cause of common death, but the mere touching of the clothes or of whatsoever other thing that had been touched or used of the sick appeared of itself to communicate the malady to the toucher.

Almost exactly two hundred years later Girolamo Fracastoro, a physician of Verona, published his *De Contagione et contagionis morbis* ('Of Contagion and contagious diseases'), a remarkable work based on Fracastoro's observation of plague, typhus, syphilis and foot-and-mouth disease in northern Italy. He defined contagion as an infection passing from one person to another, and he distinguished three types: contagion by personal contact; contagion by fomites; and contagion at a distance. 'I call fomites', he explained, 'clothes, wooden objects and other items of that sort which in themselves are not corrupted but which are capable of preserving the original seeds of the contagion and thus transferring it to others'. His use of the word 'seeds' was not significant, and his ideas bear only a superficial resemblance to the modern germ theory of disease. Nevertheless, understanding of the nature of infectious diseases increased, partly as a result of his work, and measures of segregation and quarantine became more common.

After this, very little progress was made for three hundred years, except in the case of one common and often fatal illness; puerperal fever. Puerperal fever was for centuries one of the most uncontrollable hazards of child-birth. Yet between 1795 and 1860 three doctors put forward the idea, and two of them proved in practice, that puerperal fever is a contagious disease that is preventable by means of strict but simple rules of cleanliness. Alexander Gordon was a native of Aberdeen and a graduate of Aberdeen University, and for most of his career he was a naval surgeon. For ten years, however, from 1786 to 1795 Gordon practised and taught in Aberdeen. In December 1789 an epidemic of puerperal fever broke out in Aberdeen and continued until March 1792; and in 1795 Gordon published *A Treatise on the Epidemic Puerperal Fever in Aberdeen*, a small book of some 20,000 words. The basis of his argument is a table of 77 cases of puerperal fever. The table gives *inter alia* date and period of illness, age, residence, and by whom delivered. Gordon had himself managed the delivery in 14 cases; in the remaining 63 cases midwives had been in charge, and Gordon had been called in only after the onset of the disease. Of the total of 77, 28 died, 'which proves that I have been much more successful than any other practitioner'. Gordon wrote his book in order to establish two points. First, puerperal fever was not 'owing to a noxious constitution of the atmosphere' as had been stated by Hulme, Denman and Leake, but was transmitted from one patient to the next by doctors or midwives not themselves affected by the disease: 'this disease seized such women only, as were visited, or delivered, by a practitioner, or taken care of by a nurse, who had previously attended patients affected with the disease'.[4] The table of cases supported this argument, as did such other evidence as the following:

The midwives from Aberdeen carried the infection to the Printfield, or great cotton-works, two miles from town, where a great number of lying-in women was affected; while, at the same time, the women in the neighbourhood, who were delivered by country midwives, escaped.[5]

Therefore, said Gordon, 'the cause of the Puerperal Fever, of which I treat, was a specific contagion, or infection, altogether unconnected with a noxious constitution of the atmosphere'. Secondly, he wrote in order to recommend copious bleeding as a cure for the disease: 'Bleeding and purging are the two great hinges, upon which the cure of the Puerperal Fever turns.'

Gordon's is a most distinguished little book, a work of careful observation and accurate analysis. It is unfortunate that more emphasis is placed on the method of treatment than on the means of propagation. But he states clearly that in order to prevent the disease 'the nurses and physicians, who have attended patients affected with the Puerperal Fever, ought carefully to wash themselves, and to get their apparel properly fumigated, before it be put on again'.[6] And he supports the idea – not altogether new in 1795 – that puerperal fever 'is of the nature of erysipelas'. Indeed, he not only supports it, he goes a good way to explaining it:

> The analogy of the Puerperal Fever with Erysipelas, will explain why it always seizes women after, and not before delivery. For, at the time when the erysipelas was epidemic [in Aberdeen], almost every person, admitted into the hospital of this place, with a wound, was, soon after his admission, seized with erysipelas in the vicinity of the wound. The same consequence followed the operations of surgery: and the cause is obvious; for the infectious matter, which produces erysipelas, was, at that time, readily absorbed by the lymphatics, which were then open to receive it.

> Just so with respect to the Puerperal Fever; women escape it till after delivery, for, till that time, there is no inlet open to receive the infectious matter which produces the disease. But, after delivery, the matter is readily and copiously admitted by the numerous patulous orifices, which are open to imbibe it, by the separation of the placenta from the uterus.[7]

This reveals remarkable understanding, although no knowledge of precisely what transmits the disease; in this passage Gordon refers to 'the infectious matter' but in another part of the book speaks of transmission by persons 'charged with an atmosphere of infection'.

Gordon's book was reprinted three times, and this should have given his ideas considerable currency. They did indeed exert some influence on obstetrical and medical practice in the following fifty years, although not as much as their clarity and value might lead one to expect. They were reinforced many years later, in 1843, when Oliver Wendell Holmes published a pamphlet entitled *The Contagiousness of Puerperal Fever*. Holmes is principally remembered as an essayist and man of letters, but he was by profession a doctor and became Professor of Anatomy at Harvard in 1847. His pamphlet was based on a wide knowledge of the medical literature of France (where he had studied) and Britain as well as of the United States, and he laid much emphasis on the work of Gordon. Holmes made no original discovery, but he marshalled the evidence and restated the case: it was the medical attendants themselves who were the carriers of infection. His views attracted little attention until they were attacked in the 1850s by two of the most eminent obstetricians in America, one of them C.L. Meigs who had already distinguished himself by opposing the use of anaesthesia in child-birth Meigs, like many others, took it as a personal insult to be told that he was a carrier of the very disease he professed to combat; and he preferred, he said, to attribute deaths from puerperal fever to 'accident, or providence, of which I can form a conception, rather than to a contagion of which I cannot form any clear idea, at least as to this particular malady'.[8] Holmes saw perfectly well that his opponents were not so much arguing with him as defending their injured vanity, and in his reply he took up this point:

> Let it be remembered that persons are nothing in this matter; better that twenty pamphleteers should be silenced, or as many professors unseated, than that one mother's life should be taken. There is no quarrel here between men, but there is a deadly incompatibility, and exterminating warfare between doctrines. . .[9]

Holmes was an eloquent and an urbane writer, and by the 1850s he occupied a distinguished position in American medicine; but he was unable to convince many of his contemporaries.

Gordon does not seem have known about bacteria, and Holmes also make no reference to what could properly be called a germ theory of infection. This is likewise true of Ignaz Semmelweiss, who independently, in Vienna in the 1840s, solved the problem of how to prevent puerperal fever. Semmelweiss was an assistant in the obstetric section of the General Hospital at Vienna, which was organised in two divisions. In the first of these the patients were attended by medical students under instruction, and in the other they were attended by pupil midwives. The overall deathrate was appallingly high, averaging in the region of five to ten per cent of pregnant women admitted. Semmelweiss observed, however, that this general average concealed two peculiarities, one familiar and one seemingly unique. What was familiar was that the figures varied a great deal from month to month, sometimes reaching as high as 20 or even 30 per cent. More surprising, the mortality in the division where patients were attended by medical students was invariably much higher than in the other division. For the years 1841–6 Semmelweiss found the rates to be 9.92 per cent in the former compared with 3.38 per cent in the latter, a difference of a factor of three. Semmelweiss was a keen pathologist, and he divided his time between the wards and the post-mortem room, which was only too well supplied with cadavers. He realised that there were two problems — what caused puerperal fever? Why was the death rate much higher in one division than in the other? — and that if he could solve one he would probably have solved the other. The cause of puerperal fever, however, in spite of the work of Alexander Gordon and Holmes, was not known in Vienna. Some said that it was due to epidemic influences, others that it was an acute specific fever like scarlet fever or smallpox, others that it was the same disease as erysipelas. As for the difference between the two divisions in the Vienna hospital, it was variously held that the male students were rougher than the pupil midwives, that the vitality of mothers in the presence of male students was undermined by modesty, that the very fabric of the male students' division — the walls, windows, floor-boards and beds — was inhabited to a peculiar degree by some unknown *materies morbi*. 'All this reduced me', Semmelweiss wrote, 'to such an unhappy frame of mind as to make my life unenviable. Everywhere questions arose; everything remained without explanation; all was doubt and difficulty. Only the great number of the dead was an undoubted reality.'[10]

In 1847 one of Semmelweiss's colleagues died of septicaemia resulting from a cut to his hand whilst making a post-mortem examination. Semmelweiss recognised to his astonishment that the disease that had killed his colleague was identical with puerperal fever. And he deduced that in all cases the cause was the same, that is to say, infection transmitted from a dead body. This deduction perfectly explained the difference between the mortality figures in the two obstetric divisions, because where the mortality was higher the women were attended by students who had often come straight from the dissecting room; and they had not washed their hands. It also explained the fact that in cases of easy labour puerperal fever was uncommon, but in cases of prolonged labour, or in those with complications, where several medical examinations were carried out, many women died.

Semmelweiss therefore put forward his 'doctrine' that infective material from a dead body was the only cause of puerperal fever, and he at once reduced maternal mortality in Vienna by insisting that everyone passing from the dissecting room to the wards should wash his hands in what was the best antiseptic known at that time, chlorine-water or chlorinated lime. Shortly afterwards he gave his explanation a more correct form, and taught that puerperal fever was caused by decomposed animal organic matter without regard to its origin, whether it came from a dead body or from a living person affected with a disease that produced decomposed tissue.

By means of one simple regulation, based on observation and logic, Semmelweiss rediscovered the solution to a major medical problem.

He proved his case, as Godlee says, 'conclusively to impartial minds'.[11] But although he saved many lives he did not convince many physicians. Why was this? No doubt the very simplicity of his explanation told against it. Those who wanted to believe in atmospheric, telluric or cosmic influences must have felt let down – diminished – by such a mundane proposition. Also, it was easy to carry out in a perfunctory and inadequate way the precautions which Semmelweiss recommended and then to claim that a 'trial' of his method had produced no favourable result. And the fact that Semmelweiss was a man of no great social position and had shown republican sympathies in 1848, the 'year of revolutions', did not prejudice his superiors in his favour. (Even Virchow, 'the greatest of all pathologists', poured scorn on Semmelweiss and his ideas.) Another factor that prevented the acceptance of Semmelweiss's 'doctrine' was his own failure to put it forward calmly and clearly. For these and perhaps other reasons Semmelweiss made no great and immediate impression on the world. When in 1885 Lister visited Budapest, where Semmelweiss had latterly worked, and whose discoveries Lister had confirmed and explained, his name was not even mentioned.

These improvements in medical practice that very few physicians adopted did not depend on fundamental knowledge of bacteria or on analysis of the causes of disease; and this may have been their most serious weakness. By 1850 few reasonably well-informed persons in scientific circles were unaware that bacteria existed, but the relation – if there was a relation – between bacteria and disease was quite another matter. The first steps towards a better understanding were taken by a Frenchman, Pierre Bretonneau. In 1821 Bretonneau discovered that diphtheria is a communicable disease caused by a specific germ responsible for the formation of a false and often fatal membrane in the respiratory tract. Bretonneau's recognition of diphtheria as a specific disease distinct from other inflammations of the throat was a valuable contribution to medicine. But what mattered far more, as Dr Barry Wood has pointed out, was his generalisation of this result, the fact that is to say, that he proposed:

the general theory that different diseases are due to different specific causes. This doctrine of etiological specificity, first enunciated in the 1820s, is now so firmly established that it is hard for us to imagine how it could ever have been doubted. Yet its acceptance by the medical profession was extremely slow, partly because Bretonneau's own writings did not make it sufficiently clear. Not until the closing decades of the nineteenth century did it finally become recognised as a cardinal principle of clinical medicine.[12]

Bretonneau's ideas were advanced by the researches of an Italian public servant, Agostino Bassi. Bassi was interested in microscopy, and he devoted many years to a study of the infectious disease called muscardine, which is fatal to silkworms. After twenty years of patient investigation, Bassi was able to show in 1835 that muscardine is caused by a minute fungus, and he described the several paths of transmission of the contagion. Moreover, he understood and commented upon the significance of his discovery:

> This production of mine ought to interest not only the breeder of silkworms, but also all the cultivators of the natural sciences, it being capable, perhaps, of removing some of the many anomalies which the doctrine of contagions in general presents. . . Not only am I of the opinion that the contagions, such as variola, petechia, pest, syphilis etc. are produced by vegetable or animal parasitic entities, but also that many, not to say all, of the cutaneous diseases are due to the same cause — that is, that these also are generated and maintained by the said vegetable or animal parasitic entities of different species; and I am also of the opinion *that some ulcers, though deep,* if they are not caused, are at least maintained, and for a long time, by parasitic entities, and that even gangrene is caused by such entities.[13]

In this remarkable passage the suggestion is for the first time made that gangrene might be due to 'parasitic entities', although it is notable that Bassi considered that these might be either 'vegetable or animal'. He also realised the importance of sterilisation, observing that in the process of inoculation 'the germs of a contagious disease' might be transmitted from one patient to the next on the point of a needle, and that what was therefore wanted was

> for the inoculator to carry with him . . . a small lamp . . . and having lighted this and made the first inoculation, the point of the needle that is employed is passed for three seconds, or three beats of the pulse, into the midst of the flame of the little lamp, then the second inoculation is at once made with the same needle, and so on from inoculation to inoculation. . . Whatever may be the species of contagious germ that has become attached to the wounding needle, it is

quickly destroyed by passing it into the said flame.

This, which sounds so ordinary today, was very extraordinary in 1835, so much so, indeed, that not very much attention was paid to it by practising physicians.

Also in the 1830s important work was published on the processes of fermentation and putrefaction. In 1837 Theodor Schwann clearly showed that putrefaction was caused not by the air but by something in the air which could be removed by heating. His results, however, were considered to be inconclusive. As regards fermentation, this was thought of as a purely chemical process. When it was proposed that fermentation is a vital process consisting of the action of yeast cells upon whatever chemical substances are present in the material undergoing fermentation, the general reaction was one of disbelief. The argument was relevant to medicine because it was often held that disease and fermentation were similar processes. If it could be shown that fermentation was caused by the introduction of a living organism into a host, this would strengthen the view that disease could be caused in the same way.

By the middle of the century opinion, even expert opinion, was thoroughly confused.[14] Many understood that medical science faced two closely related questions of the highest importance: were diseases caused by micro-organisms entering the body, having originated elsewhere? If the answer was in the affirmative, were specific diseases linked to specific micro-organisms? Micro-organisms had been found to exist, and it was arguable that they caused at any rate some diseases. But rival theories suggested that the onset and development of disease was a chemical fermentation-like process in which some vaguely defined self-reproducing particles of organic matter either multiplied, or catalysed an alteration in the normal chemistry of the body and thus gave rise to the development of poisonous secretions; or that disease occurred when bioplasm degenerated into living particles which were 'disease germs', quite distinct from micro-organisms, but, like them, 'capable of growing and multiplying rapidly when placed under favourable conditions'.[15] Neither of these two theories was necessarily opposed in every respect to the true germ theory. What was, without question, completely opposed to that theory was the idea of the spontaneous generation of organisms and hence of disease. And even in the 1860s it was the spontaneous generation school that dominated opinion — 'a school', as was stated in the *British Medical Journal* in 1864 'which probably embraces the great majority of medical practitioners and the whole of the "sanitary" public, [which] teaches that sundry disease poisons are constantly being generated *de novo* by the material conditions which surround us'.[16]

Such was the state of knowledge when Joseph Lister began the study of medicine, and such were some of the long-established beliefs that he had in due course to overcome. It is no doubt important that from his childhood he was in contact with scientific minds, often of a high order. His father was a prosperous wine merchant, who in his leisure hours made important discoveries in the field of optics which led to his being made a Fellow of the Royal Society. He was also a good Latin scholar, with a sound knowledge of French and German, and he knew many of the eminent scientists of the day. Young Lister thus grew up in a well-to-do home (Upton House in East London, now derelict) with books, ideas, conversation and enjoyment. For many generations his family had been Quakers, and this gave to his education and to his personality (he was as a boy cheerful and 'full of spirits') a serious but not a gloomy cast.

In 1844, at the age of 17, Lister entered University College, London, which was then the only institution in England that could be attended by those who wished to pursue the study of medicine and who were not members of the Established Church. Before starting medicine he read for an Arts Degree, in the midst of his studies he contracted small-pox and then, in 1847, suffered a nervous breakdown. During his recovery he went for a holiday to Ireland, and while he was there his father wrote him a letter which gives some indication both of the nature of the illness and of the close and sympathetic relation that existed, and that continued, between father and son:

> . . . I can hardly forbear expressing to thee the pleasure with which I look back to our cheerful parting, in connexion with the very interesting and tender interview thou hadst with thy dear mother and me before it. I have compared it to the sunshine after a refreshing shower, following a time of cloud — and I trust the remembrance of our conversation may be permitted to dispel from thy thoughts some phantoms of the dark — that thou will become fully aware of what is certainly true — viz that the things that sometimes distress thee are really only the result of illness, following too close study — and also that it is *indeed* a mistake following *from the same cause*, to believe thyself required to bear burthens on account of the states of others, while in fact thou hast to suspend even the pursuit of thy own proper avocations. And believe us, my tenderly

beloved son, that thy proper part now is to cherish a pious cheerful
spirit, open to see and to enjoy the bounties and the beauties spread
around us. . .[17]


Once more in good health, Lister began the study of medicine in
1848. At least two of his teachers were distinguished men. Wharton
Jones, Professor of Ophthalmic Medicine and Surgery, who was once
publicly spoken of by Jenner as 'one of the greatest Englishmen who
ever lived', was in fact a Scotsman whose 'small stature, peculiar manners, outrageously Scotch accent, and modest and retiring disposition'[18]
somewhat limited both his influence and his recognition. Yet Wharton
Jones made important discoveries concerning both the circulation of
the blood and — possibly significant in the light of Lister's later work —
inflammation. Lister's other distinguished teacher was William Sharpey,
Professor of Physiology. Sharpey, along with some others, has been
called 'the father of modern physiology', apparently for no better
reason than that he was the first to give a special course of lectures on
this subject. He was a graduate of Edinburgh, and had subsequently
studied both clinical and operative surgery at Paris. He was an outstanding teacher and a close friend of James Syme, a fact which was to
prove important in shaping Lister's career.

Lister took his degree in medicine in 1852. He had already done
some microscopical and experimental research work, almost certainly
under the influence of Wharton Jones and Sharpey, and the results
were published in the *Quarterly Journal of Microscopical Science* in
1853. But before becoming a practising surgeon — which he had always
intended — he wished to gain more experience, and Sharpey advised
him to go to Edinburgh for a month and then to visit the Continent and
see what was being done in the medical schools there. Thus Lister came
to Edinburgh in the autumn of 1853 and into immediate contact with
James Syme.

Lister was a well-qualified and unusually well-educated young doctor
of 26. Syme was 54 years old, certainly the most distinguished surgeon
in Britain and perhaps in Europe, and it was Lister's extreme good
fortune to come under his direct influence at the very beginning of his
career. From the outset, Syme treated Lister with special kindness and
consideration, and a friendship grew up between the two which was to
last until Syme's death in 1870. Soon after his arrival in Edinburgh,
Lister was given the opportunity to assist Syme with private operations
and simultaneously was set to work in the Royal Infirmary. In 1854

he became, in effect, assistant-consultant to Syme, enjoying the unusual privilege of deciding for himself which of the cases admitted at night he should operate on. He became, in fact, very closely identified with Syme's work, defending some of Syme's views in the *Lancet* and at one point sending to that journal weekly summaries of Syme's lectures. From the beginning Lister greatly and rightly valued this close and sympathetic contact with, as he expressed it, 'an acute and comprehensive mind working upon an experience of upwards of thirty years'.

Lister had early shown a special interest in pathology and physiology, and in Edinburgh he continued a line of research in which he had previously engaged. His object was to understand, as far as possible, the process of inflammation – a topic of prime importance to one who lectured on systematic surgery – and unlike almost all previous workers in the field he concentrated on the preliminary and not on the more advanced stages. Moreover, he appreciated the reasons why he, a surgeon, should engage in this kind of fundamental research. When theory, he wrote, as

at the present day ... is allowed such free scope, and is permitted to attack the most time-honoured rules of practice, we stand in peculiar need of the beacon light of correct pathology, to enable us to steer a safe course amid the various conflicting opinions which assail us.[19]

His observations were made mostly on the frog's web ('having got a frog from Duddingstone Loch . . . I proceeded last evening to the investigation'), and his first paper in the series describes the composition of the involuntary muscular tissue and its remarkable capacity for extension and contraction. The principal paper, read before the Royal Society in 1857, is simply entitled *The Early Stages of Inflammation*, and the main section discusses the effects of irritants upon the circulation of the part to which they are applied. Lister also deals, in the conclusion of his paper, with the mechanism of counter-irritation, stressing that 'disabled tissues' may recover, if not subjected to too severe or protracted irritation, and that their recovery 'is accompanied by a restoration of the vital fluid to the healthy characters which adapt it for circulation'. There is no reference in these papers to the observation or existence of bacteria.

It is impossible to miss the significance of these experiments, both as an indication of Lister's approach to medical problems and as a clue to his character. Few surgeons began a career in the 1850s with fundamental research; fewer still would have written of it, as he did, 'I am now really doing work'. In a short time he traced the process of inflammation, as he himself said, 'from the beginning in I believe a more satisfactory way then it has ever been traced before', and his results were obtained 'by the very simplest experiments neatly executed'. The coagulation of the blood was a problem that excited a great deal of interest at the time, and it is not surprising that Lister took an interest in it. He may or may not have fully understood its enormous significance. But what is singular is the way in which he set about investigating the fundamental problems that underlay it. Moreover, like a true scientist he found joy in the process of discovery; 'I often uttered involuntary exclamations of delight during the time'.

In 1860 Lister moved from Edinburgh to Glasgow. He had published eleven research papers, had contributed the article on *Amputation* to Holmes's *System of Surgery* which first appeared in 1861, enjoyed a growing international reputation, and was locally regarded as a skilful operator 'with a marked leaning towards conservative, as opposed to brilliant, surgery'. Above all, he was 'distinguished for his modesty and transparent honesty'.[20] During his early years in Glasgow he was a good deal occupied with work on the abdominal aorta and aspects of the excision of the wrist, but he continued his studies on the coagulation of the blood, and delivered an important paper on the subject before the Royal Society in London in 1863. In this paper he again stressed that coagulation results from blood coming in contact with 'ordinary matter', and that contact with unhealthy tissue has the same effect. How living tissue prevented clotting he could not explain. It must be due, he thought,

> to the operation of mysterious but potent forces, peculiar to the tissues of living beings, and capable of reversing the natural order of chemical affinities; forces which I suspect will never be fully comprehended by man in the present state of his existence, and the study of which should always be approached with humility and reverence.[21]

This is not, in any way, the language of modern science, but the accuracy of Lister's observations has never been questioned, and his attitude to knowledge is one shared by the greatest scientists of all ages.

As time passed, Lister's interest in inflammation and suppuration seems, if anything, to have increased, and these subjects figured prominently in his lectures. Then, in 1865, Dr Thomas Anderson, Professor of Chemistry at Glasgow, drew Lister's attention to the work of Louis

Pasteur. Pasteur is one of the great figures in the history of science, and in the 1850s he was already famous; as early as 1856 his work on crystallography had led the Royal Society to award him the Rumford Medal. Pasteur was a chemist. And it is therefore understandable that a manufacturer of beet-root alcohol, who encountered technical difficulties in his plant in the 1850s, should appeal to Pasteur for help; the latter forthwith abandoned pure chemistry and began, in 1856, a series of investigations that were to have profound consequences for the welfare of mankind.

The essential question was, what is the nature of fermentation? Attempts to find an answer to this question had been made before 1800, and by 1850 it had been shown by several workers that yeast cells grow and multiply, and as they do so turn sugar into alcohol. In short, fermentation is an organic or vital process, and not simply a chemical one. The truth of this answer, unfortunately, was denied by two of the greatest chemists of the time, von Liebig and Helmholtz, who held that fermentation is a species of slow combustion; and their views were the accepted opinion when Pasteur began work on the subject.

In succession, he studied the better-known varieties of fermentation. He observed yeast cells grow and multiply while sugar turned to alcohol, and he noted that the yeast plant assumes different shapes while wine ferments. He found organisms, 'ferments' he called them, of another kind in milk going sour with the production of lactic acid. He isolated some of these organisms, and by introducing them into a container of fresh, boiled milk, caused souring to occur. He was able to show that because ferments are different, an albuminous sugar solution can be converted into a number of different products by the addition of different ferments. What matters is the metabolism of the organism involved. 'This theory explained the facts in a way that Liebig's theory never did.'[22]

Pasteur thus proved that fermentation depended upon minute organisms, in fact, upon various types of cocci and long slender bacilli. He did not know all the details; but he did know that he had discovered the possibility of anaerobic life, that is to say, of life which flourishes not in the presence of oxygen but in its absence. This discovery reinforced the old and familiar view that there was much in common between fermentations, putrefaction, and disease, and raised once again the vexed question of spontaneous generation. Did the minute organisms which caused all these changes — in, say, a bottle of milk, or a piece of meat — did they come from within, or from without? In order to settle this question Pasteur filled some flasks with a putrescible liquid, and sealed the mouths of the flasks while the liquid was boiling. He set the flasks aside for observation.

> The organic putrescible matter was there; a conjunction of the necessary elements of life could presumably take place and evidence itself in putrefaction of the fluid. It did not take place. There was not the slightest change, and on the flasks being broken open and the fluid microscopically examined no signs of germs or other life could be detected. Why not? Because, said Pasteur, the germs in the air were prevented from getting to it. He plugged a tube with cotton wool and drew air through it. The cotton wool became black with the dust which it filtered from the air. He added a fibre of the blackened wool to a flask. The liquid in it soon showed signs of putrefaction.[23]

Pasteur's opponents were not convinced. After all, the cotton wool fibre itself was organic matter and might, therefore, itself be the source of what was needed, within the flask, for the creation of life. So Pasteur took a new set of flasks, filled them as before, and then heated and turned down the necks. Air could reach the liquid, but dust, moving only in a downward direction in perfectly still air, could not. The fluid in the flasks did not decay. But, said the opposition, how can the air be so thick with germs that putrescible matter exposed to it always is affected? On this theory the air, everywhere, is full of germs; there is no such thing as fresh, germ-free air, which is absurd. In reply, Pasteur filled a number of flasks with boiling liquid, and sealed them hermetically. He then opened them in several locations. Twenty were opened on a country road near Arbois; eight developed putrefactive changes. Another twenty were opened on a hilltop some 2,500 feet high near Salins; five developed putrefaction. Pasteur wanted to repeat the experiment aloft, in a balloon, but had to be content with the Mer de Glace. Opened here, only one flask showed putrefaction. Finally, another twenty flasks were opened in a crowded room, and all developed putrefaction. The proposition that germs existed in the air more or less in proportion to the dust that it might be expected or observed to contain was, as far as possible, proven. And along with this proof was the proof, as far as it could be obtained, that spontaneous generation was a chimera. Speaking at the Sorbonne in 1864, and having in front of his audience four flasks of sterilised broth, four years old, he spoke as follows:

I point to that liquid and say to you, I have taken my drop of water from the immensity of creation, and I have taken it full of the elements appropriate to the development of inferior life. I wait, I watch, I question it, asking it to repeat, before my eyes, the marvel of erection. But it remains silent, silent ever since I began the experiment years ago; silent because I have kept it away from the germs in the air, kept it away from life . . . Never will the doctrine of spontaneous generation recover from the mortal blow of this simple experiment.

Nor did it recover; although one might add that Pasteur's persuasive command of language played an important part in its demise.

Lister discovered Pasteur's work in 1865 through reading the *Comptes Rendus Hebdomadaires,* the weekly publication of the *Académie des Sciences.* He was particularly impressed by Pasteur's demonstration that the organisms producing fermentation and putrefaction are carried on specks of dust floating in the atmosphere, and that these organisms can be destroyed by heat, or trapped by filtration through cotton wool, or held off by having to pass upwards through a narrow passage. Equally important to him was the idea that the particles of dust are plentiful in crowded, busy rooms, but relatively absent in remote, 'clean' places. And he noted also Pasteur's demonstration that some substances, such as blood and urine, are devoid of micro-organisms, and remain indefinitely without decomposing if stored in previously sterilised vessels.

It was a saying of Pasteur that in the activity of observation 'chance favours only the mind that is prepared'. This applies equally to Lister's appreciation of the researches of Pasteur. In his paper, *Recherches sur la Putrefaction,* published in 1863 and read by Lister in 1865, Pasteur begins by saying that the problem of putrefaction derives its interest from a desire to understand the nature of disease. In spite of this, medical men showed little interest in Pasteur's work, although in 1864, in a paper read before the British Medical Association at Cambridge, Spencer Wells pointed out that the experiments of Pasteur had 'a very important bearing upon the development of purulent infection'. It was left to Lister, however, to draw exact conclusions. When Pasteur wrote that some micro-organisms could cause putrefaction deep in the putrescible fluid, obtaining oxygen from the compounds of small stability decomposed by their own vital activity, while others lived upon the surface, obtaining their oxygen directly from the air, it must have occurred to Lister that the failure of irritated or injured tissue to maintain the flow of blood might be caused by micro-organisms. In the case of a wound, where tissues were necessarily irritated and injured, micro-organisms could enter and, in conditions of low vitality, multiply; putrefaction would then be almost inevitable. On the other hand, if the skin was unbroken germs could not enter and putrefaction could not occur. Pasteur's observation that there were micro-organisms in the air, along with his experiments relating to degrees of impurity in the air, seemed to suggest that the air was the principal or sole carrier of germs. Pasteur realised, however, that germs are also carried on the surface of many solids and within many liquids, and are therefore present on hands, clothing, linen, bandages — on anything that has not been sterilised. But this point Lister did not at first fully appreciate.

Nevertheless it was Lister's genius to see how one of the causes of death — spreading and uncontrollable suppuration — could be checked through Pasteur's demonstration of the nature of decomposition; for he already knew — as he had taught for some years at Glasgow — that 'the occurrence of suppuration in a wound under ordinary circumstances, and its continuance on a healthy granulating sore treated with water dressing, are determined simply by the influence of decomposition'.[24] What could be done in the laboratory to prevent putrescible matter from decomposing by preventing the entry of germs into a flask could surely — no doubt in a different way and to a lesser extent — be repeated as regards the entry of germs into surgical wounds in a hospital. As Lister himself expressed it over 30 years later: 'All efforts to combat decomposition of the blood in open wounds were in vain until Pasteur's researches opened a new way, by combating the microbes.'[25]

In his first paper on antisepsis published in five issues of the *Lancet* between March and July 1867, Lister began by comparing 'the frequency of disastrous consequences in compound fracture' with the absence of decomposition and consequent febrile disturbance and possibly death in three other types of case: simple fracture; puncture of the lung by a fractured rib without external wound; and small wounds. He pointed out that in this last type of injury,

if the coagulum at the orifice is allowed to dry and form a crust, as was advised by John Hunter, all bad consequences are probably averted, and, the air being excluded, the blood beneath becomes organised and absorbed, exactly as in a simple fracture.

Serious illness in compound fractures was due to decomposition of the blood and other organic substances, of which the 'essential cause' had been shown by Pasteur to be in the activity of 'germs of various low forms of life' existing in the atmosphere. The problem, therefore, was to neutralise the activity of these germs in a wound, and to prevent their entry if possible.

To prevent the occurrence of suppuration, with all its attendant risks, was an object manifestly desirable; but till lately apparently unattainable, since it seemed hopeless to attempt to exclude the oxygen, which was universally regarded as the agent by which putrefaction was effected. But when it had been shown by the researches of Pasteur that the septic property of the atmosphere depended, not on the oxygen or any gaseous constituent, but on minute organisms suspended in it, which owed their energy to their vitality, it occurred to me that decomposition in the injured part might be avoided without excluding the air, by applying as a dressing some material capable of destroying the life of the floating particles.[26]

All that was necessary, he wrote, 'is to dress the wound with some material capable of killing these septic germs . . . yet not too potent as a caustic'. This was 'the antiseptic principle'.

Knowing that carbolic acid had been used as a disinfectant in order to get rid of the stench from the sewers in Carlisle, Lister obtained some of this dark, malodorous fluid, used it to clean a wound, and then applied a piece of lint, soaked in the acid, as a dressing, covered by a slightly larger piece of thin tin or sheet lead in order to prevent evaporation of the acid. The blood and carbolic acid combined to form a crust or thick paste, of which the antiseptic properties were renewed from time to time by painting some more of the indiluted carbolic acid on the outer surface, after removal of the metallic plate. This was the first antiseptic dressing, and it was a large step in the right direction. Lister soon discovered, however, that he could attack septic germs within the wound

by introducing the acid of full strength into all accessible recesses of the wound by means of a piece of rag held in dressing forceps and dipped in the liquid. This I did not venture to do in the earlier cases; but experience has shown that the compound that carbolic acid forms with the blood, and also any portions of tissue killed by its caustic action, including even parts of the bone, are disposed of by absorption and organisation, provided they are afterwards kept from decomposing.[27]

Moreover, he had scarcely introduced the idea (in March 1867) of using lint dipped in carbolic acid as a dressing than he abandoned it (at any rate in the case of larger wounds) in favour of 'a paste composed of common whitening (carbonate of lime) mixed with a solution of one part of carbolic acid in four parts of boiled linseed oil'[28] (September 1867), laid over a piece of rag dipped in the same solution, and covered with a sheet of block tin. This paste, to be changed daily as long as any discharge continued, served 'as a reservoir of the antiseptic material', and resembled a poultice.

Lister dealt in the last section of his paper with the treatment of abscess, where, 'as a general rule, no septic organisms are present'. The plan adopted was to place a piece of carbolised lint over the part to be operated on some time before the incision was made, to dip the knife in carbolic solution, and to make the incision 'under the protection of an antiseptic rag' which allowed 'the evacuation of the original contents . . . with perfect security against the introduction of living germs'.[29] As with compound fractures, the wound was covered with a piece of block tin over a layer of antiseptic putty 'about a quarter of an inch thick . . . the antiseptic rag used in opening the abscess being removed the instant before'. This dressing was to be changed 'methodically' every 24 hours. The results of the treatment, Lister reported,

are such as correct pathological knowledge might have enabled us to predict. The pyogenic membrane has no innate disposition to form pus, but does so only because it is subjected to some preternatural stimulus. In an ordinary abscess, whether acute or chronic, the original cause that led to suppuration is no longer in operation, and the stimulus that determines the continued pus formation is derived from the presence of the pus pent up in the interior. When an abscess is opened in the ordinary way this course of stimulation is removed, but in its place is substituted the potent stimulus of decomposition. If, however, the abscess be opened antiseptically, the pyogenic membrane, freed from the operation of the previous stimulus without the substitution of a new one ought, according to theory, to cease to suppurate. . . Such, accordingly, is the fact.[30]

In this first article Lister gave a careful description of eleven cases. He could not claim complete success; one patient had died and two others had contracted hospital gangrene, one of these recovering only after amputation of the infected limb. Nevertheless, eight successes out of eleven consecutive cases in one hospital, and that a notoriously unhealthy one, was a signal achievement. In the 1860s it was astonishing ('startling' is the word used by Godlee) that a patient admitted with 'compound fracture of the leg: with a wound of considerable size and accompanied by great bruising, and . . . great swelling' should, eight days later, be eating and sleeping well, and the limb be daily diminishing in size. Inevitably, a great deal of interest was aroused. Astonishment was general, not unmixed with incredulity. With abscesses, especially, Lister's success ran counter to so much experience. 'For years afterwards many who had not seen Lister's practice or obtained similar results themselves positively did not believe that his account of it could be accurate.'[31]

A month later, in a paper read before the British Medical Association in Dublin, Lister made two further points. Probably in response to criticism, he drew a sharp distinction between suppuration due to decomposition and suppuration due to the action of chemical substances such as carbolic acid. He emphasised that the appearance of pus under an atiseptic dressing was harmless:

carbolic acid stimulates only the surface to which it is first applied, and every drop of discharge that forms weakens the stimulant by diluting it. But decomposition is a self-propagating and self-aggravating poison. . .[32]

In this paper he also indicated that the antiseptic method could be applied equally well to the treatment of surgical wounds, although he was not yet satisfied that he had found, in detail, the best procedure in such cases. He did not mention the fact that, four months previously, he had made the first application of his new principles to a surgical wound; removing a deep tumour from the arm of a man 'accustomed to a bottle of port every day after dinner; not a very pleasant patient to have to do with'. The operation and recovery were a great success; 'nothing could have been more satisfactory'.[33]

Two years later Lister devised and published a further important application of the antiseptic principle in surgery. Until his time, all ligatures, made of silk or thread, were liable to cause suppuration. They were therefore cut with their ends hanging out of the wound so that they could act as a drain, to be pulled out at a later stage when they had ulcerated through the artery to which they were applied. They were thus a frequent cause of 'secondary haemorrhage' or diffuse suppuration. Lister realised that silk or linen thread contained in its interstices putrefactive germs, and that these were the cause of degeneration of the arterial wall, suppuration, and possibly haemorrhage. He therefore steeped silk thread for two hours in strong liquefied carbolic acid before use. This was not entirely successful, and he turned to catgut, which had sometimes been used for ligatures. Used in experimental work on animals, Lister found that the catgut was absorbed by the living tissue too quickly, and that when moist it became so soft and slippery that a knot in it would not hold. In a series of experiments carried out during 1869, Lister established that catgut seasoned with age and soaked for a long period in a mixture of liquefied carbolic acid and oil could serve as a safe antiseptic ligature. 'Catgut', he wrote, 'manufactured from the small intestine of the sheep, may be had at a very low price, from the thickness of a horsehair upwards'.[34]

In the following years, indeed, it is hardly too much to say, until the end of the following decade, Lister continued to develop his system. The principle remained the same; but ideas were introduced, modified, discarded. He had a laboratory in his house, and there he endlessly investigated and experimented. In 1870 he became concerned that his practice of changing the dressing daily might allow 'a single drop of serum' to be exposed 'even for a second to the influence of septic air', and that as a result 'putrefaction would be pretty certain to occur'. The difficulty of guarding against this risk had been, he thought, 'a serious drawback to the treatment'.[35] The solution he devised was to spray with a syringe, using a one-in-forty solution of carbolic acid, the surface of the wound from the moment that the dressing was removed until another antiseptic covering took its place. Secondly, he now sought to protect the wound from continuous irritation by carbolic acid. He still advised the injection of a strong solution of carbolic acid into the wound initially, the 'transient irritation' thus caused being of no account compared with 'the abiding influence' of putrefaction. But he now recognised that the continual action of carbolic acid on tissue was both destructive and unnecessary. Once more he used simple fracture ('which you cannot too often call to mind if you wish to keep your ideas clear and right upon this subject') as the model to be approximated:

> if you remember how the severe and contused internal wound, with the interstices of the mangled tissues loaded with extravasated blood, recovers quickly and surely under the protection of the unbroken integument, it is plain that all that is required in an external wound

is to guard against the disturbing influence of external agency. The injured tissues do not need to be 'stimulated' or treated with any mysterious 'specific'; ALL THAT THEY NEED IS TO BE LET ALONE. Nature will then take care of them: those which are weakened will recover, and those which have been deprived of their vitality by the injury will serve as pabulum for their living neighbours. Now, of all external agencies the most injurious by far is putrefaction, and this, above all, we endeavour to exclude. But a substance employed with this object, if sufficiently potent to destroy the life of the putrefactive organisms, cannot fail to be abnormally stimulating to the exposed tissues; and these must be protected from its action if the wound is to progress exactly like a subcutaneous injury.[36]

The problem was, how to devise what Lister called a 'protective', 'unstimulating in its own substance and impervious to carbolic acid', which could be placed between the wound and the carbolised dressing. (He must have surprised many of his colleagues when, in 1870, he remarked, 'Of all those who use antiseptics in surgery, I suspect that I apply them least to the surface of the wound.'[37]

The original dressing, little more than a crust of blood and carbolic acid, had already been abandoned. The putty dressing, reliable but inconvenient, was discarded after a short time. A 'cerate plaster', devised early in 1868, was too brittle. A lac plaster, produced soon afterwards, was too sticky, but was at once modified so as to overcome this disadvantage. The modified lac plaster was in regular use into the 1870s, but Lister was now in search of 'a perfect protective', unstimulating, insoluble, supple, and inexpensive. The answer he came up with was oiled silk, 'obtainable at any druggist's shop', and brushed over with a mixture of one part of dextrine, two parts of powdered starch, and sixteen parts of cold watery solution of carbolic acid. Soon afterwards, he became dissatisfied with the lac plaster which he used beneath the protective, and began to look for a dressing which, unlike the lac plaster, would freely absorb the discharges from the wound. This change of direction was made because the plaster dressings, besides being difficult to make and use efficiently, retained some discharge from the wound and thus kept the wound and the surrounding skin damp and even sodden. There were alternatives. Oakum was used by some surgeons as an antiseptic dressing, absorbing well and yet retaining its antiseptic properties; but it was dirty, smelly, and sticky. Lister set out on yet another series of experiments to find the ideal dressing, this time an absorbent one, and after much laborious work in the realms of applied chemistry he came up with carbolic acid gauze. This consisted of a muslin gauze, reasonably cheap, sufficiently porous and not too flimsy, impregnated with an antiseptic mixture of resin diluted with paraffin and treated with carbolic acid. A complete dressing consisted of a pad of gauze eight layers thick, plus an impermeable layer near the top. The antiseptic gauze was eminently successful and was used for many years. It had, however, two defects; the carbolic was slightly caustic to the wound, and from the time it was applied the gauze lost some of its effectiveness due to evaporation of the carbolic. In 1889, after another series of experiments lasting over five years, Lister produced the double cyanide of mercury and zinc gauze, and this remained for several decades the most satisfactory antiseptic gauze in existence.

In 1871 Lister introduced the carbolic acid spray. Deeply impressed by the presence in ordinary air of millions of particles of dust and invisible micro-organisms, and believing that a high concentration of pathogenic organisms was the rule, Lister sought to surround not only the wound itself but the entire operating table with an antiseptic atmosphere in which germs would be unable to survive. His proposal was to annihilate them in a mist of carbolic acid vapour. At first only a small hand-spray was used. But soon a foot-operated spray was introduced, and before long this gave way to the 'steam spray', a piece of apparatus capable of enveloping the patient and all those engaged in the operation 'with a more or less dense, damp, and pungent mist'. Needless to say, this aspect of antiseptic surgery was far from popular. Sometimes the spray would not start, and sometimes, having started, it stopped in the middle of an operation. Sometimes it would not adjust properly, and the surgeon's hands, and the patient, were drenched with carbolic acid which, although supposed to be a weak solution, could turn fingers white and numb. All those present inhaled the vapour, which made some people sick, and when operations were performed in a room illuminated by gas or lamps, or heated by an open fire, the combustion could decompose the chloroform vapour, setting free acrid chlorine gas which immediately affected the nose and throat of everyone present, and the eyes of everyone except the patient, who had the advantage of being unconscious. In spite of these very objectionable features, the spray was used all over the world for several years. Criticism was persistent, and when a distinguished German surgeon finally wrote a paper in 1880 with the arresting title *Fort mit dem Spray* (Down with the Spray), its use began to decline. But Lister continued to defend it, and to use it, until 1887.

During these years Lister also worked on the problem of the drainage of wounds. Drainage was more important with the antiseptic treatment than without it, because the antiseptics which were in use irritated the cut surface and produced more serious effusion than was normal. Lister fully recognised this difficulty; 'it is impossible', he wrote in 1875, 'to exaggerate the importance of drainage tubes'.[38] He adopted the idea of using rubber drainage tubes, introduced by Chassaignac in 1859, and he constantly emphasised the advantages of using rubber tubes 'from the thickness of a crow-quill to that of the little finger', several in a large wound. He also continued to elaborate the minor precautions that were always necessary: 'If a knife or other instrument, after being used during an operation, is temporarily set aside or even withdrawn for ever so short a time from the antiseptic atmosphere of the spray, it must be cleansed afresh with carbolic lotion' before being brought back into use.[39]

Thus the essentials of Lister's antiseptic system were all put forward between 1867 and 1871; but the system was under continuous development for more than 20 years. What that system, as a working practice, amounted to in 1870 differed significantly, although certainly not in principle, from what it amounted to in 1880 or in 1890. Components were added to the system, modified within the system, and, in at least one instance, namely the spray, finally removed from the system. It is therefore very difficult to describe. Merely to outline the details, which were important, would require many pages. They included, for example, the strength of the carbolic acid solution, which might vary for different purposes; the mode of its application; the make-up of the dressing, possibly many layers of material thick; its size; the frequency with which it was to be changed, which again would probably vary according to the type of wound and progress of the patient; precautions necessary when changing a dressing; placing of drainage tubes; what action to take if inflammation developed in spite of these procedures and so on. The emphasis placed on different items also changed over the years. It was and is very easy to oversimplify what Lister proposed, and his contemporaries were apt to think it all very complicated indeed. What was consistent was the theoretical foundation and Lister's attitude towards the problem he had to solve. He was, always, a pathologist as well as a surgeon, and he would have found it impossible to separate these two aspects of his work. He made as well as worked from new pathological discoveries. It was he who found that a portion of dead tissue is not necessarily thrown off by suppuration but 'serves as pabulum for the

growing element of the new tissue in its vicinity', that new tissue growing in a wound, beside a piece of bone superficially dead, could coalesce
with live tissue within the bone, absorbing the dead stratum — an
occurrence that was generally held to be impossible; that a ligature of
catgut, although seemingly remaining intact round a vessel, would be
absorbed and replaced by living tissue — 'nothing could be more beauti-
fully in accordance with all I have before made out, or more satisfactory
*practically'*. Dealing with the very principles of life, Lister was so
much more than an operating surgeon that it was inevitable that most
of his fellow surgeons should fail to understand him.

In 1883, at a time when he had been developing his system for 16
years and was to continue to develop it for another ten, he described
seven cases of fractured olecranon (the bony point of the elbow) which
he had operated on with complete success. In the course of his description he made some general observations which illustrate very well both
his point of view at a time when his system had few converts still to
make, and his simplicity, directness, earnestness, and nobility of character.

I have referred to a case of ununited fracture of the olecranon where
eighteen surgeons had been previously consulted. I trust no one here
will suppose that I mentioned this circumstance for the purpose of
glorifying myself. I mentioned it in order to emphasise what I
believe to be the truth, that by antiseptic means we can do and are
bound to do, operations of the greatest importance for our patients'
advantage, which, without strict antiseptic means, the best surgeons
would not be justified in recommending. How wise these eighteen
gentlemen were in counselling against operative interference, provided they were not prepared to operate strictly antiseptically, I
think we must be all agreed. As regards the operative procedure in
that case, it was of the most simple character; any first year's student could have done the operation exactly as well as myself; and,
therefore, I trust I shall not be misunderstood by its being supposed
that I came here to extol my own skill. That which justified me in
operating in that case was simply the knowledge that strict antiseptic treatment would convert serious risk into complete safety.

I should have liked, if time had permitted, to have said a few words
as to what seem to be the essential points as regards antiseptic treatment. If I say any words at all now, they will be exceedingly few. I
should just like to make this remark, however, that nowadays anti-

septic tretment is not a very complicated business, either in theory or in practice. First, as to theory, we do not require any scientific theory to enable us to believe in antiseptic treatment. You need not believe in the germ theory at all; if you are not convinced of the truth of the germ theory of putrefaction and of septic agencies generally, no matter whatsoever with reference to antiseptic practice. All that you have to believe is that there are such things as putrefaction and other septic agencies, and that our wounds are liable to these, and that they are very pernicious, and that these things come from without, and that we have the means of preventing them by various chemical agencies. That is all that we require; and I think that anybody who knows the present state of surgical practice must admit these to be truisms. It has sometimes been a great grief to me to think that, because gentlemen are not convinced of the truth of the germ theory out and out, therefore they lay aside antiseptic treatment altogether. And then as to practice; it is not a very difficult thing to wash your hands in a carbolic solution, and have your instruments in their carbolic solution for a quarter of an hour before you operate. It is not a very difficult thing to wrap around the limbs a suitable envelope of antiseptic material. What I believe to be one of the most important things of all is . . . always when we change a dressing, invariably first to cover the wound with something pure; not to wash the surrounding parts with antispetic solution, and then, after that has been done, put a dressing on the wound; but before we begin to defile the lotion at all, put on the wound what is pure, and last thing of all, wash the surrounding parts, which, though they look the same to our eyes, are different *toto caelo*. The edges of the dressing are septic; the wound, if it is as it ought to be, is aseptic. I have known such a thing, for instance, as for a gentleman, in dressing a stump after amputation of the thigh, to wash the perineum with a rag dipped in the carbolic lotion one in forty; and then, having so washed the perineum, immediately to squeeze the rag over the wound. Gentlemen, that makes you laugh; but I assure you these are the kind of things that are constantly going on, and disasters happen in consequence; and gentlemen with whom things go wrong invariably say that with them everything has been perfectly done — a thing which, for my part, I am always loathe to say.

I am not likely to have many more years of active surgical work; and I have felt that when you, Sir, gave me this opportunity, it was my duty to speak what I believe to be the truth; for I felt it to be a grievous thing that patients should be hurried out of their lives, or deprived of usefulness of limbs, simply for want of sufficient earnestness with regard to the endeavour to obtain complete exclusion of septic agencies from wounds, according to our present lights and our present knowledge.

Gentlemen, I thank you most heartily for your cheers; for there was a time when such remarks might have met with a very different reception.[40]

When Lister spoke these words he was a man of 56. There were still many modifications he was to make to his system, and some of his colleagues still to be convinced of its value. His remarks are therefore, so to speak, an interim statement — unlike most of his contemporaries, he had little belief in finality. But this manner towards people and his approach to problems changed little over the years, and the sentences quoted give a very good indication of both.

No one questions that Lister had an enormous influence on the practice of surgery in the second half of the nineteenth century. But precisely what was it that he discovered, or invented, or devised? His contribution was multiple; over the years item was added to item, although everything was directed to a single end. But partly because what he tried to do could be done in several ways, it may seem — as it did seem to some contemporaries — that he was not always in the forefront of progress, that other men were achieving as much as he, without introducing as many complications or attracting as much attention.

Lister made great advances in surgery in two ways, ways which can never, when significant, be entirely separate, and which in his case were always very closely intertwined. First, he and he alone perceived in the mid-1860s the medical significance of the work of Pasteur. This was an achievement of theory: to deduce that the decay of a putrescible fluid exposed to airborne germs was precisely analogous to the decay of tissue in an open would may seem, in retrospect, not very difficult; but the fact is, that only one man made this deduction. The information on which the deduction was based was readily available. Pasteur's work was well known; he was famous; he was not slow in publishing his results, and in 1864 he had explained to a very large, fashionable and scientific audience at the Sorbonne that 'putrefaction is determined by living ferments'. In the previous year, even, he had said that 'all my ambition was to arrive at a knowledge of the causes of putrid and contagious diseases'.[41] This is entirely understandable; the idea that fermentation and disease might be connected was an old one. But if other men in the mid-1860s took the hint, none of them can have understood the medical implications in the complete way that Lister did. It is true that he was peculiarly well placed to do so, for he was a surgeon who was also an experimental scientist, and this combination of interests was essential and unusual. But the flash of insight that turned the light of Pasteur's work upon the dark corridors of surgery achieved in a moment what might have been the slow understanding of decades.

Secondly, Lister devoted half a lifetime to devising and improving the means to make the germ theory of disease serviceable in surgery. He had to make the theory, so to speak, applicable, to realise its enormous potential for saving human life. So he devised the tools and invented the practice of antiseptic surgery. This too was a tremendous achievement. It was partly a technical matter — the use of carbolic acid, the lac plaster, the catgut ligature, the spray, the double cyanide gauze — but at almost every step he had to depend on his own laboratory research which in its turn depended on scientific, usually chemical or bacteriological, understanding. Surgery is a rather special activity, because it is at the same time, in the language of Whitehead, a profession and a craft. A profession, according to Whitehead, consists of activities which are subject to theoretical analysis and which can therefore be modified by conclusions resulting from that analysis, whereas a craft is no more than a traditional activity subject to modification only by the trial and error of individual practice. Surgery is clearly both, and Lister was a master of both. Even if the germ theory of disease had been pioneered by someone else, his practical contributions, worked out with great skill in the laboratory, would have ensured him an outstanding place in the history of surgery. It is true, of course, that he made mistakes. Most obviously, he greatly and persistently overestimated the likelihood that 'ordinary' air would contain dangerous numbers of pathogenic organisms, and he underestimated the capacity of healthy tissue to fight back. These mistakes were made because laboratory research at that time did not provide the necessary knowledge. But according to the latest information available at the time, Lister's system was for a quarter of a century the best that could be devised to reduce post-operational mortality caused by germs. That system, in its general conception, its technical equipment, and its detailed application, was his invention.

156    *Germs, Inflammation and Antisepsis*

## Notes

1. Quoted in W.B. Wood, *From Miasmas to Molecules* (New York, 1961), pp. 14–15. This and the following paragraph draw heavily on Dr Wood's excellent little book.

2. B. Marten, *A New Theory of Consumptions: More Especially of a Phthisis or Consumption of the Lungs* (London, 1720). The quotation in the text is from Wood, *From Miasmas to Molecules*, pp. 16–17.

3. Quoted in Wood, *From Miasmas to Molecules*, p. 18.

4. A. Gordon, *A Treatise on the Epidemic Puerperal Fever in Aberdeen* (London, 1795), p. 63.

5. Ibid., p. 65.

6. Ibid., pp. 98–9.

7. Ibid., pp. 56–7.

8. Quoted in B.J. Stern, *Society and Medical Progress* (Princeton, 1941), p. 192.

9. Ibid., p. 193.

10. Quoted in R.J. Godlee, *Lord Lister,* (Oxford, 1924), p. 139.

11. Godlee, *Lord Lister*, p. 140.

12. W. Barry Wood, *From Miasmas to Molecules*, p. 24.

13. A. Bassi, *Delmal ael seqno, clacino, muscardine* (Lodi, 1835), p. 9.

14. There is an excellent discussion by J.K. Crellin, in F.N.L. Poynter (ed.), *Medicine and Science in the 1860s* (London, 1968).

15. L.S. Beale, 'Microscopical Researches on the Cattle Plague', Appendix to *Third Report on . . . the Origin and Nature of the Cattle Plague* (HMSO, 1866), pp. 129–54.

16. *British Medical Journal*, vol. II, (1864), p. 356.

17. Godlee, *Lord Lister*, p. 16.

18. Ibid., p. 17.

19. *Collected Papers of Joseph Lister*, vol. I, (June, 1857), p. 209.

20. Godlee, *Lord Lister*, p. 82.

21. Lister, *Collected Papers*, vol. I, p. 69.

22. C. Singer and E.A. Underwood, *A Short History of Medicine* (Oxford, 1962), p. 331.

23. G.T. Wrench, *Lord Lister, His Life and Work* (London, 1913), p. 94.

24. Quoted in Godlee, *Lord Lister*, p. 179.

25. Lister to Dr G.H. Edington, December 1902, quoted in D. Guthrie, *Lord Lister,* (1949), p. 56.

26. *Lancet*, vol. II, (21 September, 1867), p. 353.

27. Ibid., p. 353.

28. Ibid., p. 354.

29. Ibid., 27 July, p. 95.

30. Ibid.,

31. Godlee, *Lord Lister*, p. 188.

32. *Lancet*, vol. II, (1867), p. 354.

33. Letter to his father, 22 April 1867, quoted in Godlee, *Lord Lister*, p. 195.

34. *Lancet* (3 April, 1869), p. 455.

35. *Lancet* (3 April, 1870), p. 440.

36. Ibid.

37. Ibid.

38. *Lancet* (27 March, 1875), p. 435.

39. Ibid.

40. Quoted in Godlee, *Lord Lister*, pp. 483–5.

41. Ibid., p. 175.

# 5 THE FIGHT FOR ANTISEPSIS

Considering that Lister's 'antiseptic system' did more than anything before or since to reduce the risks of surgery and to increase its scope, and considering also that it was not a hit-and-miss affair but was based on sound scientific experiment and reasoning, why did it take so long for the medical profession in Britain to accept it? Lister first described the principles of antiseptic surgery in a series of papers in the *Lancet* which appeared between March and July 1867 and which were entitled *On a new method of treating Compound Fractures, Abscesses, etc. with observations on the Conditions of Suppuration.* In the following ten years he spoke on the subject at several surgical congresses and published numerous articles and communications in learned journals. Yet at the International Medical Congress in London in 1881, attended by many of the most distinguished medical men and scientists in Europe, including Huxley, Koch and Pasteur, what was called 'Lister's method' was ridiculed by one of the best-known surgeons in England, and declared by another to be no improvement on what it aimed to supersede. By the middle of the 1880s such hostility had vanished, and not to admire Lister and to follow his methods was to be old-fashioned, dangerous and even absurd. But why did it take the medical profession in England approximately 15 years to adopt what a great German surgeon called in 1881 'this greatest advance that surgery has ever made'?[1]

One man alone can make a discovery, but several are needed to make a revolution. If surgery in the second half of the nineteenth century was to be changed, it had to be changed by the medical profession, or at any rate by the bulk of the surgeons who were members of that profession. Lister made a great discovery; or, it might be more accurate to say, he utilised in an entirely novel way a great discovery in bacteriology made by another person. He also developed the equipment and the techniques needed to exploit his new understanding. But before there could be much in the way of practical consequences, the experts of the day, or at least a large and influential number of them, had to be convinced that the new procedures were in some extensive and practical sense 'better' than the old. The adoption of new ideas depends on the one hand upon the persuasiveness of the manner in which they are presented and on the other on the receptiveness of the audience to

157

which they are addressed. What is new must be clearly explained, its significance and importance pointed out (where it fits in, what old ideas it replaces, what its consequences are likely to be), it must be presented tactfully and not in scorn of what is currently believed, and it may have to be said over and over again. As far as the audience is concerned, criticism and resistance are the probable reactions, even to the most persuasive case. Men do not welcome new ideas that require them to think afresh, to change their habits, reorganise their professional or business procedures, instruct their assistants in different routines, and admit that what they have previously believed or practised or taught to others is not, after all, the final solution. Moreover, presentation and reception are not distinct and separate in a closed society such as medicine. New ideas are to some extent judged — to some extent must be judged — by the professional standing of those who put them forward. Within a reasonably small and very exclusive group — and medicine was making itself increasingly exclusive in the middle decades of the nineteenth century — each individual occupies a distinct position of more or less authority and credibility, based on the general judgment of his previous utterances and achievements. Hence even a very strong case and well-presented argument may find few supporters if it is put forward by someone who, for quite separate reasons, does not occupy a position of high regard within the society to which he and the ideas he is arguing for belong.

As the advocate of a new principle in surgery, Lister laboured under several disadvantages. In the first place, his personality was against him. Among those who knew him best he inspired immense admiration, immense respect, and, subordinate to these, an affection that seems almost always to have been careful and restrained. Upon his wife he depended enormously for support and encouragement, and after she died Lister was never to the same extent an active force in the world. Apart from her, he seems to have known intimately and to have confided in only his father and his father-in-law, James Syme. To other men he was kind and considerate, and with a few he shared some of his problems and enthusiasms; but to the great majority of men he was grave, earnest (earnest even for a Victorian) reserved and unapproachable. Perhaps the only person who was not related to him and who yet could claim to know Lister at all well was Sir Hector Clare Cameron; and his son, who as a boy encountered Lister occasionally at his father's house and a little elsewhere, subsequently wrote as follows:

In an age when a strict formality was the rule, he was more than usually formal, precise and reticent. At this distance of time any attempt to get behind a reserve which was impenetrable to his contemporaries is not likely to be very successful. . .

His movement was always slow and pensive. . . He was in many ways shy and reserved. When agitated or embarrassed, his repressed emotional state showed clearly in an increase of the slight stammer which he never completely lost, a twitching of the corner of his mouth and of his eyebrows and a mounting colour. . .

Lister was no weakling. From his early days he was a leader of men. He held strong opinions and he expressed them strongly. He took quick decisions and he adhered to them. He was an innovator and his innovations were all his own. Yet he was gentle, shy and in some things diffident. With all his greatness and strength there was always a certain clinging quality about him. He loved to share with those who were close to him his secret plans and projects, to sense their approval in success and to seek their sympathy in failure. . .[12]

It would be an understatement to say that Lister did not make friends easily; he hardly made them at all. He was not, like Simpson, open, cordial, ebullient, brushing difficulties aside, a good companion and a noisy opponent who enjoyed a fight. No less than Simpson he was determined to succeed; his human sympathy, probably, was no less; but he pursued his ways privately, almost by stealth, and such a man is likely to receive but a cool reception from his colleagues when he attempts to engage their support. Perhaps he tended too readily to believe that reason of itself would prevail.

Added to this, Lister was neither an eager nor a skilful contravertialist. In his first two papers he set out to explain the essentials of his system. But the title of his first paper on antisepsis, as Cameron has pointed out, was not well chosen. He was announcing to the world, as he seems very well to have realised, a discovery of major importance, namely, that suppuration is caused by decomposition of the blood, and that this decomposition results from the activity of minute living organisms suspended in the air, 'which by developing in a decomposable substance determine a change in its chemical arrangement, analogous to the fermentation of sugar under the influence of the yeast plant'.[3] This being the essential point, it was not helpful to describe his work as 'a new method of treating compound fractures, abscesses etc.' and then simply to add the words 'with observations on the conditions of suppuration'. True, Lister's initial work had been done almost entirely on compound fractures. He may have chosen to concentrate on this class of wound because the treatment of compound fractures led, in a very large number of cases, to suppuration and death, and therefore success in such cases could not be dismissed as accidental or trivial. But to emphasise the class of case was to obscure the generality of the principle. He seems soon to have realised his mistake, for the title of a paper given by him at Dublin a few months later was *On the Antiseptic Principle in the Practice of Surgery*.[4]

These two early statements attracted a great deal of attention. The first, dealing with the principles of antiseptic treatment as well as with eleven cases in considerable detail, was spread over four issues of the *Lancet* and amounted — quite exceptionally for that journal — to about 14,000 words; the second had the advantage of being delivered to the annual meeting of the BMA, held in August 1867 in Dublin. Reaction was mixed. The *Lancet* appreciated, to some extent, the importance of what Lister claimed: 'If Professor Lister's conclusions . . . should be confirmed . . . it will be difficult to overrate the importance of what we may really call his discovery'.[5] And the *Lancet* grasped the very important and indeed momentous fact that Lister's practice was founded on fundamental research into physiology and bacteriology:

> Professor Lister's idea of surgery is a truly Hunterian one. He is not a surgeon who can be content to consider his art as consisting in the skilful use of the knife. He claims, equally with the physician, the right to take assistance from physiology and chemistry.

But this point was not widely appreciated. A far commoner view was that Lister's new method was just another in the long series of proposals for improvement in the dressing of wounds. Everyone agreed that this was an important subject. The commonest system was that of water-dressing, which amounted to keeping the wound constantly covered with cold wet cloths; Syme, in 1863, changed over to metal sutures and pads of dry lint; another plan that found favour in the early 1870s was to leave the wound completely uncovered and not dress it at all. Part, but only part, of what Lister proposed could be seen as an alternative to these plans; and for this reason, perhaps, many misunderstood his ideas or underestimated them from the first.

Another serious difficulty arose because many people saw Lister's early work as being concerned with 'the power of carbolic acid in compound fractures'; and the idea that what Lister proposed was essentially the use of carbolic acid as a disinfectant in surgical operations in general soon become widespread. Numerous surgeons related how they had 'adopted carbolic acid'; one even referred to 'the curative influence attributed to carbolic acid by Professor Lister'.[6] To many people for a good many years Listerian surgery was simply 'the carbolic acid treatment', or 'the putty method'. It has to be said that at least once Lister used the former phrase himself. In a letter to his father written in June 1867 he states:

> My visit to Mr Syme was a most satisfactory one. He said 'no one can say that the operation [I propose to perform] does not afford a chance', and he also alluded to the carbolic acid treatment of wounds (which he has been trying with much satisfaction) as depriving the operation of danger.[7]

Carbolic acid quickly began to be used in all sorts of ways. It was variously applied, but the majority of surgeons found 'the multiform plasters described by Mr Lister'[8] to be more trouble than they were worth. Much the commonest plan was to dab the wound with a solution of carbolic acid diluted sometimes one in ten, sometimes one in 40, sometimes one in a 100. The fact that carbolic acid unless well diluted was apt to burn the skin and cause suppuration was frequently complained of. Lister claimed in 1870 that some people had taken him to say 'if you do but apply carbolic acid freely to a wound you will prevent suppuration', whereas he had 'all along pointed out' that carbolic acid, being a stimulating substance, would of itself induce suppuration; but this was not made clear in the early articles, in one of which he had even advocated 'the energetic application of the antiseptic agent'.[9] As a result, carbolic acid was misused. At King's College hospital a patient under Mr Wood almost succumbed to the ill-effects of carbolic acid, but recovered as a result of 'a thorough draught of air kept up by means of a fire and open windows, and the sulphate of magnesia administered internally, with wine, brandy, quinine and good diet'. In Birmingham, Lawson Tait, who was a surgeon of real ability, interpreted the method, in at least one case, to mean 'continuous irrigation with carbolic water (one in 50) for five weeks'; the patient did not do well. Some surgeons, on the other hand, altogether rejected the idea of using carbolic acid; from Guy's it was reported that Mr Birkett 'finds his cases do very well on the usual plan'.[10] At St Bartholomew's, however, Mr Holmes Coote found carbolic acid 'useful', although 'he does not approve of Mr Lister's method, which he considers meddlesome'.[11] At Middlesex Hospital the chief question was thought to be whether carbolic acid was better than choice of zinc, but it was agreed, and reported, that carbolic acid did no good sprinkled on the floor. A few surgeons in London and elsewhere were using lint dressings or lac plasters before 1870, and there was some appreciation of the fact that great care was needed if the dressings were to serve their antiseptic purpose. But attempts at a careful following of Lister's advice were comparatively uncommon.

That the proposed new antiseptic system consisted of little or nothing more than splashing a solution of carbolic acid on surgical wounds was a gross misunderstanding that at once undervalued Lister's work and opened the way to allegations that he was not suggesting anything new. The principal effort to belittle the antiseptic system in this way was made by Sir James Simpson. It has often been stated, although seemingly without evidence, that Simpson was the author of a letter which appeared in the *Edinburgh Daily Review* in 1867 and which asserted that whereas Lister had used carbolic acid in surgery for only a few months, 'it has been employed for years past by some continental surgeons, in the same cases and complications as those for which Mr Lister had availed himself of its services'. The letter further stated that a Dr Lemaire had published 'a thick volume on the subject' in 1865[12] in which there was discussed 'at great length' the use of carbolic acid in numerous fields including surgery; and the writer went on to say that Dr Lemaire

> points out very fully and elaborately its power of destroying microscopic living organisms, germs, or sporules — adduces the opinions on these matters of Pasteur, Helmholtz, Schultze, Schwann, etc., and shows its utility in arresting suppuration in surgery, and as a dressing to compound fractures and wounds.

This letter was noticed in the *Lancet,* and Lister at once wrote a short and fairly sharp reply. Lemaire's book, he observed, 'does not appear to have attracted the notice of our profession, or produced, in the country where it was published, any practical effects such as might have been anticipated from its alleged contents'.[13] Visitors to his wards from continental hospitals had never expressed the slightest doubt that his system was entirely new, not in using carbolic acid but in the methods of its use. At Dublin, he said, there had been a feeble attempt to decry the antiseptic system as useless; now an attempt was being made to impede its progress on the ground that it was not original. Two weeks later he wrote again, to say that he had now been able to examine a copy of Lemaire's work, and that 'the principles and practice which he mentions are such as sufficiently to explain the insignificance of the results'.[14] And once more he pressed home the familiar points: surgeons 'must not expect carbolic acid to act like a charm'; it must be employed 'only by the light of sound pathology, and strict attention to practical details'.

Whoever wrote the *Edinburgh Review* letter, Simpson certainly shared its author's opinions. He had said at the Dublin meeting that Lister's use and application of carbolic acid was not original, and in November 1867 he came forward with a long article in the *Lancet* which established both his failure to understand the antiseptic method and his opposition to it. Writing in his usual oratorical style, Simpson was nothing if not emphatic. Appealing to several French authors, principally Lemaire, he declared that 'the very same theory, the very same practice, and the very same means of reducing that theory to practice, have all been worked out and published on the continent years ago'.[15] Not content with saying (correctly) that the use of carbolic acid as a disinfectant in surgery was not new, Simpson sought to show that Lemaire had anticipated Lister in every point and had gone far beyond him. According to Simpson, Lemaire knew that decomposition was a result of the multiplication of minute organisms, and had shown that carbolic acid, 'even in very small doses, has the power of preventing and arresting any such decomposing effects . . . by at once and immediately [sic] destroying the life of the organisms themselves'. Lemaire had also shown, wrote Simpson, that carbolic acid was useful in treating scrofulous ulcers, burns, venomous bites, gangrene ('the ravages of gangrene, he says, have often thus been stopped as if by enchantment'), inflammation, gonorrhoea, carbuncles ('where its action, he avers, is marvellous, probably from its containing living organisms, which he thinks he has detected with the microscope'), whooping cough, angina, dyspepsia, and numerous other maladies. In short, Lemaire had thought of applying carbolic acid or some similar preparation to nearly everything, 'leaving Professor Lister very far behind him'.

As an indication of Simpson's style of thought and of his approach to scientific problems this is a very revealing article. Only two weeks earlier Lister had advised the profession not to expect carbolic acid 'to act like a charm'; now they were assured that it worked or might work 'as if by enchantment', because someone else had said so. When Simpson lent his very considerable authority to denying Lister's originality and discrediting his antiseptic system he was presumably sincere; but he was not disinterested. During the 1860s his fertile mind had conceived the idea that instead of using silk ligatures, which decomposed and often caused suppuration in wounds, haemorrhage could be arrested by means of needles passed beneath the vessels. This method Simpson called acupressure, and it was adopted in some places in Scotland with occasional success. It is not unreasonable to suppose that Simpson disliked Lister's proposals at least in part because antiseptic surgery was a rival to acupressure. In the last few hundred words of his article he states the case for acupressure as the best method to obtain the closure of wounds by first intention and without suppuration.

This intervention by the famous discoverer of chloroform anaesthesia must have had some effect. Lister replied briefly, saying that he forbore to comment on the allegations, 'having already endeavoured to place the matter in its true light without doing injustice to anyone'.[16] Some letters followed in support of Simpson, but also some in support of Lister. Whatever his influence, Simpson had not stopped antiseptic surgery in its tracks. During 1868 an increasing number of surgeons in London and elsewhere experimented with antiseptic methods, and in some hospitals it became customary to employ carbolic acid dressings of one sort or another. Lister, 'that distinguished, original, and philosophical surgeon', as one writer to the *Lancet* called him, may have felt that reasonable progress was being made. Then, towards the end of 1868, Simpson wrote a long article that began the hospitalism controversy.

This controversy has probably never received the attention it deserves. Simpson's proposal, that all large hospitals be knocked down and replaced by thousands of small iron sheds, has usually been treated as best forgotten; a silly idea founded on bad arguments, a sudden adventure into a field that he knew very little about, the final random spark (he died, worn out, twelve months later) of an enormously enterprising but erratic genius. Such an assessment seriously misunderstands both the origins and the consequences of Simpson's last contribution to medicine.

The essence of his view was that hospital diseases resulted largely from the design and management (or rather the misdesign and mismanagement) of hospitals. Far from striking out this idea more or less by chance in 1869, Simpson had put it forward quite clearly 20 years before. In his Report on the Edinburgh Royal Maternity Hospital for 1844–6[17] he stated that the 'febrile and inflammatory attacks' suffered by many patients during convalescence were due to the conditions surrounding them, in particular to overcrowding and bad ventilation.

> Everyone acquainted with hospital practice . . . is well aware of the great liability among the patients to febrile and inflammatory attacks whenever the wards are overcrowded; and in no practice is this more visible than in midwifery. . . I have often stated and taught, that if our present medical, surgical, and obstetric hospitals were changed from being crowded palaces, with a layer of sick in each flat, into villages or cottages, with one, or at most two patients in each room, a great saving of human life would be effected.

During the 1850s and 1860s, in his lectures in Edinburgh, Simpson continued to lay stress on the contagious nature of disease and on the consequent need for cleanliness in hospitals and among doctors and nurses. In 1867 he again took up the theme in public, speaking in Belfast to the National Association for the Promotion of Social Science. Maternal mortality, he said, was higher in hospitals than in private homes; did 'the same law' hold good for surgical patients?

> To what extent are hospitals, as in general and at present constituted, banes or blessings? And how can they be changed so as to convert them from the former to the latter?. . . The man laid on the operating table in one of our surgical hospitals is exposed to more chances of death than the English soldier on the field of Waterloo.[18]

Doubtless the surgeons and hospital managers whom Simpson sought to persuade would have found his arguments more acceptable if he too had been a surgeon, and not merely an obstetrician.

In any case, assertion was not enough. To support his position Simpson had to produce good evidence, or reasoned arguments, or both; and this was what he tried to do in the spring of 1869. His case for change, first put forward in the *Edinburgh Journal of Medicine* for March and June 1869, was arresting and at first sight impressive. He had collected figures ('an imposing agglomeration of figures' the *Lancet* called them) which seemed to show that in rural private practice mortality after operations was far less than in large urban hospitals; and that there was, in fact, a gradient of risk, the larger the hospital the greater the rate of surgical mortality, the smaller the hospital the smaller the rate of mortality. In particular, Simpson drew attention to those figures which seemed to show that in rural private practice the rate of mortality after amputation through the bones of the upper and lower limbs was 10.8 per cent, whereas the mortality after the same kind of operations in large urban hospitals was 41 per cent. From this he concluded that the cause of the differences in deathrate was the unhealthier conditions in the large urban hospitals, conditions which were caused, he said, by the aggregation of sick in one building, 'or, in other words, the absolute size of an hospital'. And the remedy which he proposed was the substitution of small, single-floor, moveable iron sheds for the existing three-and four-storied permanent brick or stone buildings.

Simpson's case, which he restated in no less than 22,000 words in the *Lancet* in the course of 1869 (the last instalment appeared after his death in 1870) attracted a great deal of attention. It amounted to a most serious onslaught on the existing hospital system, and caused, it was said, an immediate and serious falling off in the charitable donations upon which that system almost entirely depended. Discussion among doctors began at once — Simpson's standing in the profession ensured that — and the BMA meeting at Leeds in 1869 was largely devoted to attacking or defending Simpson's statistics and proposals. It was, after all, intolerable to find, as Sir John Ericsen put it, 'the town free from infection; the hospital saturated by it, to such an extent as to induce its own surgeons to recommend their patients not to enter it, to compel them to refrain from operating'.[19] The next two years were to a considerable extent occupied with a long discussion about the possibility or impossibility of preventing pyaemia and other 'hospital diseases' from obtaining a permanent hold in the wards of any large hospital.

The figures upon which Simpson founded his case would hardly impress a modern beginner in statistics. His first and by far his most important table was the following:

Proportionate mortality of limb amputations in Great Britain as regulated by the size of the hospital and the degree of aggregation or isolation in which the patients are placed.

| | | |
|---|---|---|
| 1) In hospitals of 300 beds to 600 | 1 in 2½ | die |
| 2) In hospitals of 100 beds to 300 | 1 in 4 | die |
| 3) In hospitals of 25 beds to 100 | 1 in 5½ | die |
| 4) In cottage hospitals under 25 beds | 1 in 7 | die |

5) In isolated rooms in country
practice      1 in 9 die

These figures, according to Simpson, 'teach a lesson of vast import in relation to hospital hygiene; and yet they seem to discourse so plainly as to require no comment'.[20] He concentrated attention on the first and last lines of this table, but produced many other tables, including one based on the work of a Dr Lefort of Paris, who 'has collated the results of nearly a million women delivered in the lying-in hospitals of Europe, and nearly an equal number of pauper patients confined in their own homes', with the following results:

Of 888,302 delivered in hospitals 30,394 died or 1 in 29
Of 934,781 delivered at home  4,405 died or 1 in 212.[21]

The second of these tables had better be passed over in silence; but the defects of the first are bad enough. The returns of amputations in large hospitals quoted by Simpson were certainly imperfect, while those relating to country practice were collected by Simpson himself, from 374 doctors selected by himself, relating to amputations carried out over a period of 20 years or more. No one could regard them as a fair sample. Far more serious, Simpson completely ignored the fact that the death rate after operations is under the influence of a great number of causes, of which the most important is the nature of the cases operated on. And there was good reason to suppose that the urban mortality figures included a far larger proportion of persons who were seriously unhealthy or of low vitality than did the figures for country practice, and that the 'hospital surgeons' operated far more frequently than did their country colleagues on cases in which death was from the start virtually inevitable. Simpson also ignored the fact that death might be caused by previous disease or concomitant injury, by operative disaster, or by the want of skilled nursing and attention. His basic argument (even supposing his figures to have been right) that the death rate after amputations was a reliable measure of the healthiness of a hospital was hopelessly fallacious.

That Simpson's figures in no way established his case was pointed out in a very able series of articles by Thomas Holmes, surgeon to St George's hospital, in the course of 1869 and again in 1871. But Simpson was not easily stopped. He could not meet the statistical objections – which were in fact unanswerable – but he kept pointing out that some figures seemed to support his argument, he introduced new

and often irrelevant information, and he evaded or seemed to mis-
understand serious objections made by his critics – for example, 'Mr
Holmes proposes to obtain acquaintance with the *causes* of death after
amputation, without even enquiring into the *rates* of death.'[22] This
was typical Simpson argument, and no doubt it bamboozled many
people. But although his statistics were silly and his logic defective,
his proposals were another matter. No doubt it was impracticable
to pull down or abandon all large hospitals and substitute thousands
of iron sheds with one or two rooms in each, or even hundreds of
cottage hospitals. But it was not so easy to dismiss the argument
that hospital diseases – even if they  did occur after operations in
private homes as well as in hospitals – had something to do with
hospital hygiene, and that hospital hygiene was poor because of 'the
aggregation of invalids within an hospital'. Simpson, an anti-Listerite,
maintained that disease in a hospital arose from 'the influence of
morbific contagious materials from the bodies of the inmates', or
was caused by 'inflammatory secretions', and he moreover pointed
out to 'our hospital surgeons' that

> the obstetric physicians of Great Britain generally agree, I believe,
> as to the occasional [sic] spread of puerperal fever . . . by the
> unhappy and indirect medium of the physician, nurse, etc. as well
> as by contagious miasmata. . . It is a question of contagion as well
> as a question of crowding.[23]

If this was so with puerperal fever, why not also with hospital diseases?
     Simpson's argument was thus, in the end, very confused. Was he
talking about the size of hospitals, or about 'contagious miasmata' and
ventilation, or about overcrowding, or about the spread of disease by
'physician, nurse, etc'? He failed to disentangle these separate items. He
concentrated on hospital size, which was a mistake, and then switched
to overcrowding as a cause of disease, which his statistics did not
approve. Indeed, one of their salient weaknesses was the assumption
that each size-category of hospital was occupied to the same extent.
But to offset all these defects his position had one element of enormous
strength; he knew that puerperal fever was a contagious disease, and he
knew how it was transmitted.
     It is constantly stated that Gordon, Holmes, and in particular
Semmelweiss laboured in vain, that their discovery about puerperal
fever had, at some unspecified subsequent point of time, to be rediscovered. But this is not the case. In Simpson's lecture notes for

1840[24] the analogy between puerperal fever and erysipelas is considered under five headings, as follows:

a) Contemporaneous epidemic prevalence
b) Erysipelas or puerperal fever patients
c) Attendants on erysipelas may carry puerperal fever to their
   patients
d) Attendants on puerperal fever seized with erysipelas
e) Direct innoculation of the poison

It is quite clear, from this and other passages, that Simpson had read
Gordon's book (there is a copy of it in his library in the Royal College
of Physicians in Edinburgh), that he thought it at least possible that
'the existing cause' was the same in the two diseases, and that 'propagation by Contagion' was a strong possibility. These notes were written
seven years before Semmelweiss recognised the connection between
erysipelas and puerperal fever. Secondly, it has recently been found[25]
that in a student's notes of Simpson's lectures given in 1848—49 it is
clearly stated that puerperal fever is spread by doctors and midwives.
The notes also indicate that in Scotland at least, doctors usually took
steps to prevent the spread of infection:

> there are still some violent non-contagionists who will go on after
> they have got it [puerperal fever] in their practice, until it is a sort
> of professional murder — Every man is morally bound to give up
> his practice for a time when at most two cases have occurred.

Thus Simpson knew perfectly well that puerperal fever was spread as
Gordon (and latterly Semmelweiss) stated, and he taught his students
accordingly. Nor was this knowledge confined to the lecture room.
In November 1850, Simpson published an important article entitled
*Some Notes on the Analogy between Puerperal Fever and Surgical
Fever.*[26] In this article he pointed out that both conditions were now
ascribed to 'some diseased or vitiated condition of the blood', and
that both showed the same or similar symptoms — rapid pulse, nausea,
local pains, general prostration, and at last rapid sinking. The spread of
puerperal fever, he went on, had come to be understood, at least to the
extent that few British obstetricians now doubted the efficacy of
measures

> calculated to prevent the medical practitioner or the nurse being

the unhappy medium of carrying the contagion of the disease from one puerperal patient to another . . . there exists, I believe, on record, a series of facts amply sufficient to prove this at least, that patients during labour have been and may be locally inoculated with a *materies morbi* capable of exciting puerperal fever; that this his *materies morbi* is liable to be inoculated into the dilated and abraded lining membrane of the maternal passages during delivery, by the fingers of the attendant . . . this *materies morbi* . . . seems to be the inflammatory products effected upon the serous or mucous surfaces of females who are suffering under puerperal fever, or who have died of it.

And he proceeded to point out that just as the bruised tissues of a puerperal patient were evidently receptive of contagion, so might be the bruised tissues of a patient with a surgical wound; as he put it a few months later, 'if [the cause of fever] could be inoculated [by hand] into the abraded surface of the vagina, it could be inoculated into a recent wound'.[27] The diseases were analogous; might not the method of transmission be analogous also? 'The question is perhaps a far more momentous one than the simple past neglect of it might *a priori* lead us to infer.'

The idea of the analogy was not new; it was owed to Gordon, recently supported by Semmelweiss. In Simpson's 1850 paper Semmelweiss's success in Vienna is described and two references to accounts of his work are given, one in French and one in English. Simpson — to whom Semmelweiss's conclusions cannot in any case have seemed novel — thus made no attempt to conceal his knowledge of Semmelweiss's work. He may, indeed, have been responsible for the visit to Edinburgh in 1851 of a Dr F.H. Arneth from Vienna who read a paper to the Edinburgh Medico-Chirurgical Society on Semmelweiss.[28] Later that year a discussion took place in the Society on the transmission of puerperal fever,[29] a discussion in which Simpson played the major part. He quoted Gordon as well as Semmelweiss, referred to Arneth's 'apparently incontrovertible evidence' that doctors and others could be the unwitting carriers of puerperal fever, stated that 'British accoucheurs generally have a belief in the contagious communicability of puerperal fever, and take their measures accordingly', and reiterated his conviction 'that surgeons, like accoucheurs, were occasionally the unhappy media of inoculating their patients with morbid matter, producing in them surgical fever, as in puerperal patients; obstetricians, by the same means, produced in their patients puerperal fever. He had no doubt that it would take many long years to convince surgeons of this fact.' These views did not apparently surprise the Society, and the conclusion must be that, at least among the better-informed doctors and obstetricians in Scotland and in England, the mode of the transmission of puerperal fever was understood.

This was an important advance in medicine, and it seems likely that Simpson played some part in it. As for the suggestion that hospital diseases might be transmitted in the same way as puerperal fever, this was Simpson's own. Semmelweiss reasoned from surgical fever to puerperal fever, Simpson reasoned in the reverse direction. Moreover, he stated, in 1850, that it was a 'momentous' question whether or not surgical fever was transmitted by doctors and nurses. Although a long way from antisepsis, this was, at least, a brilliant intuition; and, along with the accepted knowledge about puerperal fever, it lent weight to Simpson's campaign for hospital reform.

His argument in that campaign was confused, and his statistics a liability and not an asset. After some years the gold would be separated from the dross. But the hospitalism controversy which Simpson initiated had an immediate as well as a more remote impact. What took effect from the beginning was the general focus on poor hospital conditions as favourable to the spread of disease, and, in particular, Simpson's pleas for more fresh air and less overcrowding. When the BMA meeting at Leeds which discussed these matters was over, Syme wrote a long letter to the *Lancet,* in which he observed with characteristic coolness that 'all the copious statistics and unscrupulous statements adduced in support of [Simpson's] thesis might very well have been spared' because as long ago as the Peninsular campaign it had been established that operations, especially amputations, had far less chance of success in crowded divisional hospitals than if performed in a ditch or by the side of a hedge, where the patient possessed 'the inestimable advantage of pure air'.[30] His conclusion, however, was not that existing hospitals should be torn down but that they should not be overcrowded with beds too close together, especially with beds occupied by patients suffering from septic diseases, and that their ventilation should be improved. Better advice could not have been given. Later, in the course of the hospitalism debate, it was recalled that in 1833 Syme had advised that the newly-opened wing of the Edinburgh Royal Infirmary should be closed for several weeks in order to get rid of hospital disease and then reopened with only two-thirds of the number of patients previously admitted; this being done, the hospital remained in a healthy condition.

Oddly enough, Simpson never advocated reducing the number of beds in hospitals, but concentrated on improved ventilation. In order to prevent 'the rapid diffusion of light and aëriform bodies' and the spread of 'the exhalations, cutaneous, pulmonary etc. which emanate from each patient', he wanted all stairs and corridors to be open to the fresh air, or else each ward to be entered only from without, by means of an external staircase if necessary. These suggestions, not unlike others made at the time by Florence Nightingale, were not popular in all quarters; 'Surely nothing more ludicrous ever received the sanction of a respected name,' said Holmes. But Simpson, although not wholly right, was not altogether wrong. His case could have been better presented; but it was not worthless, and what he lacked in finesse he made up with force. Contemporaries were impressed. Even when the point had sunk in that the statistics proved nothing — 'It seems to us little more than a waste of time to count up the number of deaths after amputation or injury at any given hospital, and accept the total as a measure of its healthiness or unhealthiness'[31] — the fact was much more recognised after Simpson's campaign than before that there was some connection between hospital diseases and the design and management of hospitals. 'We maintain', said the *Lancet* towards the end of 1871, 'that these diseases, in their origin and development, depend far more upon our defective system of hospital hygiene than upon any other cause'.[32]

This lengthy controversy had an obvious bearing on Lister's work. He must have been helped by the argument that puerperal fever could be communicated by the hands of attendants and that the cause of surgical fever might in a similar way be inoculated into open wounds. But little attention seems to have been paid to this. And the main argument was against Lister, because to the extent that fresh air was the answer to surgical mortality, antisepsis, presumably, was not. The abolition of suppuration and putrefaction might be, as the *Lancet* put it, 'great objects to secure', but their abolition 'could not be regarded as providing a substitute for pure air in our hospitals'.[33] Looked at in this way, the hospitalism controversy did Lister's cause no good. On the other hand, it gave him an excellent opportunity to state the impact of the antiseptic system on the conditions in a large hospital, and this he did with a paper entitled *On the Effects of the Antiseptic System of Treatment upon the Salubrity of a Surgical Hospital.* He wrote principally to show that in the new wing of the Glasgow Royal Infirmary, erected in 1860, and which proved almost from the date of its erection disappointingly and indeed extremely unhealthy, he

had been able to reduce the death rate in amputations solely as a result
of the introduction of his antiseptic system. In 1864 and 1866 (the
records for 1865 being defective) there had been in his wards 35
amputations and 16 resultant deaths; from 1867 to 1869 there had
been 40 amputations and 6 deaths. 'In short, hospital gangrene, like
pyaemia and erysipelas, may be said to have been banished by the
antisepetic system . . . the facts recorded in this paper are of extreme
importance with reference to the vexed question of hospital construction.' There is no need, he wrote, for 'congeries of cast-iron cottages';
the unhealthiness of hospitals, small or large, is primarily if not solely
the result of 'emanations from foul discharges'.[34] Get rid of decomposing wounds and you get rid of the problem.

If this had been all that Lister made public, along with some supporting detail, the consequences for adoption of the antiseptic system
might have been favourable or even very favourable. And even as it
was, his paper caused the *Lancet* to call for a fair and crucial trial of
his methods to be made in London, where there were 'hospitals which
afforded only too good a field for testing the system'. But here, and not
for the last time, Lister's inability to state less than the whole truth as
he saw it, bluntly but in considerable detail, made enemies of some,
and distracted attention from his real message. Not content with
describing his wards in Glasgow as initially 'extremely unhealthy' he
wrote of them as 'some of the most unhealthy in the kingdom', and
then went on as follows in a passage which, although well known,
requires to be quoted in full.

At this period I was engaged in a perpetual contest with the managing body, who, anxious to provide hospital accommodation for
the increasing population of Glasgow, for which the infirmary was
by no means adequate, were disposed to introduce additional beds
beyond those contemplated in the original construction. It is, I
believe, fairly attributable to the firmness of my resistance in this
matter that, though my patients suffered from the evils alluded to
in a way that was sickening and often heartrending, so as to make
me sometimes feel it a questionable privilege to be connected with
the institution, yet none of my wards ever assumed the frightful
condition which sometimes showed itself in other parts of the
building, making it necessary to shut them up entirely for a time. A
crisis of this kind occurred rather more than two years ago in the
other male accident ward on the ground floor, separated from mine
merely by a passage twelve feet broad; where the mortality became

so excessive as to lead, not only to closing the ward, but to an investigation into the cause of the evil, which was presumed to be some foul drain. An excavation made with this view disclosed a state of things which seemed to explain sufficiently the unhealthiness that had so long remained a mystery. A few inches below the surface of the ground, on a level with the floors of the two lowest male accident wards, with only the basement area, four feet wide, intervening, was found the uppermost tier of a multitude of coffins, which had been placed there at the time of the cholera epidemic of 1849, the corpses having undergone so little change in the interval that the clothes they had on at the time of their hurried burial were plainly distinguishable. The wonder now was, not that these wards upon the ground floor had been unhealthy, but that they had not been absolutely pestilential. Yet at the very time when this shocking disclosure was being made, I was able to state, in an address which I delivered to the meeting of the British Medical Association in Dublin, that during the previous nine months, in which the antiseptic system had been fairly in operation in my wards, not a single case of pyaemia, erysipelas or hospital gangrene had occurred in them; and this, be it remembered, not only in the presence of conditions likely to be pernicious, but at a time when the unhealthiness of other parts of the same building was attracting the serious and anxious attention of the managers. Supposing it justifiable to institute an experiment on such a subject, it would be hardly possible to devise one more conclusive.[35]

Everything that Lister wrote in this paper was correct and everything was relevant. But it annoyed two sets of people. Those who had been his colleagues at Glasgow took offence at the overt comparisons between 'my wards' and 'the frightful condition which sometimes showed itself in other parts of the building'. Yet such a comparison had to be made sooner or later. The whole point of Lister's work was that it saved lives whereas older methods lost them. To make the claim, however, was to imply, or to seem to imply, that other surgeons were losing lives that might be saved; this was a serious implication, and to many it was offensive. This was a difficulty that Lister could not avoid, but he might have minimised it, and at the same time kept on the right side of the hospital managers, who were the second set of people whom his paper annoyed, had he included in it, and given due weight to, some other information about conditions in the hospital in the later 1860s. His version was that 'a shocking disclosure' — indeed several shocking disclosures — had been made about the situation of the hospital; that he had had to engage in 'a perpetual contest with the managing body' in order to prevent dangerous overcrowding in his wards; that, even so, and in spite of all he could do, he had sometimes felt it 'a questionable privilege to be connected with the institution'. The general impression was that the Glasgow hospital was an exceptionally unhealthy and ill-managed institution, although that was not precisely said and was probably not intended.

Being only human, the managers, several of whom were doctors or surgeons, were bound to react against such statements. Certainly the siting of the hospital was exceedingly bad, but when the truth about it was discovered the managers were as upset as anyone else. The words 'perpetual contest' made the attitude of the managers appear in the worst possible instead of in the best possible light. And to speak of his association with the hospital as 'a questionable privilege' was somewhat gratuitous, although there can be no doubt that the words were carefully chosen and represented Lister's sincere opinion.

The Secretary of the Infirmary accordingly published a reply[36] contradicting some of Lister's statements, severely criticising others, setting out statistics to show that mortality after amputations was less at Glasgow than at Edinburgh, and claiming, above all, that in the opinion both of the Directors and 'those of their number belonging to the medical profession'

. . . the improved health and satisfactory condition of the hospital, which has been as marked in the medical as in the surgical department, is mainly attributable to the better ventilation, the improved dietary, and the excellent nursing to which the Directors have given so much attention of late years.

Although in some respects defective, as Lister was able to show, this reply raised an extremely important and valid point which did a great deal to obscure the merits of Lister's own case. For it was indeed true, as the Secretary pointed out, that changes in the general conditions in the hospital had, at the same time that Lister introduced his new techniques, brought about an overall improvement in the health of all patients. Lister had been, to say the least of it, unwise not to acknowledge this fact; if he did not know it he should have made it his business to find out before drawing comparisons which turned out to be not quite accurate. And had he referred to this general improvement he would, of course, have mollified the managers and at the same time not made his fellow surgeons appear quite so unsuccessful in comparison with himself.

More important than this, the fact of general improvement made it impossible, on the available evidence, to disentangle the contribution made to health and recovery by Listerian techniques from that made by improved hospital conditions. In the surgical section improvement was most marked in Lister's wards; but it was open to anyone to argue that these wards had benefited more than others from the efforts of the managers — that these wards had started, so to speak, from a lower level. This argument was wrong. But it could be advanced with a show of reason that was sufficient to weaken severely the persuasiveness of Lister's case.

Nor was this all. For the fact of general improvement was a fact. There was indeed another way to improve the health of patients in hospitals and even to reduce, if only a little, the mortality after operations. Lister was not willing to recognise this. In a long reply to the letter from the Secretary, he made three points. The first — 'extremely satisfactory to myself' — was that the figures quoted by the Secretary

. . . serve to contradict, on competent authority, an anonymous statement which was made some time ago in one of the medical journals, and has been repeated *ad nauseam* in various quarters, implying that the use of antiseptic measures in the Glasgow Infirmary had led to an increased mortality. This statement, which was said to be founded upon the hospital records, I could hardly have contradicted, although it was entirely the reverse of the truth as regarded my own department, without appearing to cast a slur upon the practice of my colleagues. But I rejoice to find that, taking the results of the practice of all the four surgeons of the hospital, the death-rate during the three years of the antiseptic period has been less by fully one-fifth than during the five previous years.

Secondly, he acknowedged that the need for hospital treatment had placed the hospital managers in a very difficult position:

When speaking of the struggle [to limit the number of patients] as a contest, I intended nothing disrespectful to the managers. Each party had a laudable object in view. They desired to accommodate as many patients as possible, while I was very anxious that those who were admitted should have favourable atmospheric conditions;

and these two laudable objects were for a time antagonistic.

Had some such statement been made in Lister's original article, the issues would not have become so confused and much antagonism would have been avoided. What was now said put the record straight; but the harm done could not be entirely undone. Thirdly, Lister rejected completely the suggestion that the improved results in his wards could in the smallest degree be attributed to anything other than the antiseptic system; such an attribution 'is simply out of the question':

> As regards the ventilation of these wards, it remains precisely as it was, with the exception of a freer access of air to the back of the hospital, in consequence of taking down [a] high wall. . . As to nursing, my department was not affected by the change that occurred. . . And as to the dietary, the idea tht a mere improvement in rations would abolish pyaemia, erysipelas, and hospital gangrene, is one which would hardly enter the mind of an intelligent medical man.

All of which was no doubt true. And yet it is easy to see that in the light of all these other arguments and considerations Lister's case was entirely convincing only to those who were already convinced. A number of changes had taken place in the Glasgow hospital, and improvement had resulted. But to decide the relative importance of the several changes made was not easy, especially for those who were not on the spot. Lister's statements had about them a certain air of the absolute and the peremptory. To human fallibility and the chance of error he seemed to concede little – and indeed he did concede little. Faced with an entirely novel doctrine which made enormous claims and carried with it potentially enormous consequences, and seeing it enveloped in arguments and counter-arguments that were relevant although not essential to it, it is hardly surprising that many surgeons were inclined to believe that there was a good deal less in 'antisepsis' than Lister claimed.

Fresh trouble arose a few years later, again partly due to Lister's uncompromising attitude. In 1873 John Wood, Professor of Surgery at King's College, London, gave the address in surgery to the annual meeting of the BMA and devoted about one quarter of his time to the antiseptic system. The system, he said, had been originally developed by Lemaire in 1860, and he himself had recently experimented with various antiseptic substances and dressings, with and without 'the elaborate attempts to exclude the unpurified atmospheric air which Lister deems essential'. He had obtained, he said, good results both with Listerian and un-Listerian methods when the hospital was free of pyaemia and similar diseases, but when these diseases became present results deteriorated whatever the method used. His conclusions echoed the hospitalism debate:

> I believe that cases of recovery frequently occur under other methods, or no methods, and that at least as much depends upon the age and reparative power of the patient, the amount of blood poison formed or absorbed, and the general condition of the atmosphere, as upon any system of treatment whatever.[37]

The tone of Wood's address is judicious and many of his observations are sensible and shrewd. But again Lister responded sharply. Development of the antiseptic system, he wrote, was leading to ever greater success in preventing putrefaction in wounds, so that pyaemia and hospital gangrene had never reappeared in his 'crowded wards'; as to why Wood was unable to achieve the same results, 'of the many strangers who have witnessed my practice since his address was given, not one appears to have had any hesitation in arriving at the true explanation'.[38] This acidulous comment resulted in protest on Wood's behalf and allegations that Lister's wards contained cases of inflammation and suppuration very much like any others.

Perhaps as a result of these statements and counter-statements about what was and what was not to be found in Lister's wards, Samson Gamgee, surgeon to the Queen's Hospital, Birmingham, paid a visit to his 'old friend and fellow-student' in Glasgow, and published some clinical notes which had been checked by Lister. But he added some comments which had not been checked, and once again Lister's response was hostile and uncompromising.

Gamgee's description of the cases is careful and thorough and might have been written by Lister himself. His comments are relatively brief and may be further abbreviated as follows:

1. No detail is too minute, no time too long, for him. If the patients were princes, and if the office were rewarded with the salary of a prime minister, duties could not be discharged with more exquisite gentleness, nor in a purer spirit of scientific research, within the limits of the knowledge at hand.

2. At first advising the introduction of *carbolic acid of full strength* into all accessible recesses of a wound, in order to destroy the septic germs [1867], we find Mr Lister four years later teaching that 'in direct proportion to the *weakness of the solution used* and the smallness of its opportunity of acting on the tissues of the part, is the satisfactoriness of the result obtained, provided that the essential object of avoiding putrefaction be secured' [1871].

3. The drainage tube is more important with antiseptic treatment than without it, because the antiseptic treatment irritates the cut surface, and in the first few hours there is more serious effusion than without it.
   Lister's work is by drainage as well as by antisepsis.

4. To Pasteur Lister gives 'unflinching fidelity', and his results vary from good to 'brilliantly good'. But a theory becomes a handicap when 'made to fit all difficulties'. Antisepsis is not the only modern aid to surgery. Other surgeons rely on other dressings, on compression, suspension, ventilation.

What is needed is a thorough scientific examination of the whole question [of the treatment of wounds] discarding the fatal bias of a fixed theoretical preoccupation.[39]

These are, on the whole, very fair comments, and they are much more for Lister than against him.

Lister at once wrote a reply both brief and chilling. He hoped that readers would distinguish between Dr Gamgee's facts and his opinions. As to the statement that he entertained 'a fixed theoretical preoccupation' which was 'made to fit all difficulties', this was 'a grave charge' made publicly 'against my professional character' which he declined to discuss. Gamgee responded with a polite and reasonable letter in which he regretted that 'scientific and professional controversies are so apt to become personal' and denied that his remark about a fatal theoretical bias was a personal charge. He reiterated that a thorough examination of the whole question was called for. The inescapable although incorrect impression given by this correspondence is that Gamgee was an intelligent and highly qualified professional enquirer, whereas Lister could not separate scientific ideas from notions of his own importance and required from those who approached him only one response, total agreement.

On one further and important occasion Lister demonstrated this unhappy capacity to turn friends or potential friends into enemies.

On the eve of leaving Edinburgh for the Chair of Surgery at King's College, London, Lister addressed his students and took the opportunity, as Godlee puts it, 'of contrasting, at some length, the clinical professorships in the two cities'. His remarks included the following:

> But if I turn to London, and ask how instruction in clinical surgery is conducted there, I find that, not only according to my own experience as a London student, which I once was, but also from the universal testimony of foreigners who visit there, and then come here, it is, when compared with our system here, a mere sham. . . The magnificent opportunities of demonstrative teaching presented by clinical surgery are, to a great extent, neglected.

This appears to have been an impromptu speech, and certainly it was not a public one. Nevertheless, it was reported next day in the Edinburgh and London papers (as private speeches sometimes are) and of course caused much anger. Indignant letters appeared in the *Lancet*, and once again Lister had to reply to irate criticism. In the course of a lengthy explanation he withdrew the word 'sham', and expressed astonishment that anyone should have supposed him to be criticising individuals. He did not, he said, presume to compare himself with any other surgeon. What he objected to was the inadequate and perfunctory teaching of clinical surgery in London. He was advocating Syme's method of clinical instruction, which Lister himself had always followed,[40] and he wanted to see it adopted in London because he passionately wanted better surgical education and better surgery. A few months later, lecturing in London, Lister conceded that he might have done some individuals an injustice, and that he seemed to detect in the metropolis 'considerable changes since I was a student'. But that was as far as he would go. His surprise that many men had taken his words as reflecting on their own competence or attention to duty shows very clearly his inability to realise that the pursuit of truth in medicine was not a goal which relieved others, as it did him, of all vanity, all self-seeking, all regard to personal reputation or personal advantage. It is not exactly true that he thought of only one thing at a time, or that he was a man of one idea. Nor is it true that he had no sympathy for the feelings of others. But he seems to have thought that what was true must always be spoken. In one who is trying to persuade his fellow men, it is a most serious error.

Lister was thus not a skilful propagandist for his system; indeed, the very idea of propaganda would have been abhorrent to him. But even had he possessed all the arts of persuasion, he would have had to over-come three very serious difficulties in convincing his colleagues that they should adopt the antiseptic system. These difficulties were, first, the complexity, indeed the ever-changing complexity of what he pro-posed; second, the possibility that there were other and simpler means to the same end; and third, doubt about the germ theory.

That Lister's proposals were apt to be misunderstood has already been remarked. Often they were simplified almost out of recognition — depicted, for example, as simply involving the free use of carbolic acid. This interpretation was common until at least 1870: 'Young medical men, and the public generally, are being taught to regard this acid as a panacea';[41] 'carbolic acid . . . the latest toy of medical science, so-called'.[42] Lister himself observed that 'the publication of my first papers was followed by a very general employment' of carbolic acid, which was then given the credit for any good results achieved.[43] Some men made a more serious attempt to understand and apply the system, sometimes with even more unfortunate results. The earlier versions of the antiseptic technique were complicated and cumbersome, and even Godlee, who was Lister's son-in-law and wrote the official biography, admits that 'the early methods were not perfectly satisfactory'.[44] As the *Lancet* wrote in 1870, 'It has taken Professor Lister five or six years to bring his own antiseptic treatment to its present degree of perfection; and we have no reports of anything like similar pains being taken in any of our London hospitals . . .'[45] Many trials of 'the anti-septic technique' were made in these years, but most of them were carelessly carried out and very often the mere occurrence of suppura-tion was held to have proved the failure of the treatment. As late as 1873 Godlee had to explain yet again that 'suppuration may be caused by any abnormal stimulus whatever. . . It is the occurrence of putre-factive suppuration alone that involves the failure of the antiseptic treatment.'[46]

At least one of these 'trials' of the system can be described in detail. In 1869 one of the most distinguished surgeons of the day, Sir James Paget, 'a man devoid of jealousy and of a singularly open mind',[47] and who became President of the Royal College of Surgeons in London in 1875, announced the result in a case of compound fracture of the leg. As soon as the operation was over the wound was sealed up with collo-dion, and twelve hours afterwards carbolic acid putty was applied. Three days later, in spite of the exceptional care taken in employing the carbolic acid 'after the manner which has been so strongly recom-mended by Professor Lister . . . if not with all the skill that Professor

Lister would employ, yet with more than is ever likely to be generally used in the treatment of fractures', it was found that the limb had become 'swollen, tense, very hot, and very painful' and that the patient showed 'all the signs of very acute fever'.[48] This case is most revealing. It would be generous to describe it as a grotesque caricature of Listerian surgery. It has some of the elements, but in a hopelessly mixed-up and contradictory fashion; and it demonstrates total and absolute ignorance of the principles involved. In a letter to the *Lancet* Lister observed, with almost superhuman restraint, that 'the practice followed in this instance had very little in common with anything I have advised'. Carbolic acid was not used to cleanse the wound before operating; after the operation the wound was sealed up with collodion, trapping any putrefactive agents within; twelve hours later a superficial carbolic acid dressing was applied, and the wound again sealed. Lister's observation on this last procedure was simply to say that 'to combine collodion and carbolic acid is to do not only what I never thought of recommending, but what I should regard as objectionable, since the former would tend to obstruct the free exit of the sero-sanguineous effusion which the stimulating action of the latter would promote'.[49] And if this was how Sir James Paget understood Listerian surgery, what did less eminent surgeons think and do? In 1877 it was reported from Paris that 'the principles of Lister are so imperfectly understood by a good many French surgeons, that I had shown me at various hospitals "modifications" of his method in which everything is present except his principles'.[50] It was much the same in Britain. Even attempts to use the catgut ligature had disastrous, in one case fatal, consequences.

It is easy to understand that careless or partial or incompetent attempts to follow Lister's methods should have had bad results. But some of the critics were able and successful surgeons. One of the most remarkable of these was Lawson Tait. Born and educated at Edinburgh (he was a student of Syme, and often referred to Simpson as 'my master'), Tait came to prominence as an ovariotomist in 1872, when he was still in his late twenties. In spite of having seen 30 ovariotomies performed in Edinburgh without a single recovery, he took up this branch of surgery and in 1872 reported ten ovariotomies with three deaths. At this stage he used what he called 'Listerian precautions' but without much conviction.

My opinion of the antiseptic treatment is that its merits have been greatly over-rated, and its good results, which are quite as uncertain as those of other means, are due more to the greater care taken of the cases, and [in abscesses] to the exclusion of air.[51]

By 1880 Tait was perhaps one of the ten or twelve most famous and respected surgeons in Britain, and his opposition to antisepsis had hardened. He had now performed 100 ovariotomies. In the first 50 he lost 19 patients. in the second 50 he lost three patients. The improvement, he said, was due entirely to a change in operational method and had nothing to do with antisepsis. The results depended not on the exclusion of germs but on 'the power of vital resistance by the tissues or the condition of the patient'.[52] Ten years later he made the same point, a not invalid one, very forcefully when he wrote,

> Lister's view was 'keep out the germs and you may leave bloodclot (and other matters) to take care of themselves'. My view was and is, 'Get out all decomposable matter and you can let the germs in freely.[53]

His opposition to antisepsis was not confined to its use in ovariotomy. In 1880 he reported the 'almost uniform result' that

> wounds dressed after Lister's plan suppurated, and in many cases they sloughed; and though none of the patients died, many of the recoveries were anxious and protracted. Some of my critics said this was due to my imperfect method of using the dressings. My answer was that if the proper use of the dressings was above my limited intelligence, it was useless for general application, and that ... I would go back to the old-fashioned dry lint.[54]

Tait had a good deal of influence. Like his 'master', he was never behindhand in controversy, and as a surgeon he was without an equal for cleanliness, manual dexterity and speed. It was also important that he did not belong to the London 'establishment' but worked in Birmingham, and always showed 'a want of respect for age and authority remarkable even in Birmingham'.[55]

The success of some of those who opposed Lister, however, it might be explained, added to the bewilderment of the profession. Simple hostility was one thing. It did not much matter that a well-known surgeon like Nunneley should, as Lister put it, 'dogmatically oppose a treatment which he so little understands, and which by his own admission he has never tried'.[56] Nor was it of the first importance that the cost of the antiseptic system was exciting 'the serious consideration of the managers' of the Glasgow Royal Infirmary (and no doubt the managers of other hospitals also) in the middle and later 1870s. (In 1875 Lister thought it worth-while to explain at length how to make surgical gauze for 2d per square yard, or half the wholesale price.) But it was very disturbing that not a few surgeons claimed, apparently with justice, that without resort to antiseptic surgery they had achieved results which an earlier generation would have considered little short of miraculous. Lister's antiseptic dressing was only one of the surgical novelties of the time. Some continued with Liston's water-dressing — 'the perfection of lightness compared with a poultice; the perfection of cleanliness contrasted with ointments, often irate, sometimes rancid'[57] — but added drainage tubes, introduced by Chassaignac in France and improved by Lister; 'drainage is all that is needed to place most wounds in the most favourable condition for healing'.[58] Others favoured the new practice of doing without dressings altogether:

The 'antiseptic' method, in which every 'germ' is rigorously excluded by clouds of spray and multiplied layers of gauze, and the 'open-air' method, in which a wound is left open to all that the atmosphere may chance to deposit upon its surface, differing as they most absolutely do in the theory on which each is founded, appear, in many operations at least, to be about equally successful in practice.[59]

So said Sir Eric Erichsen, with a lifetime of experience behind him. An anonymous author listed a few rival success stories:

Mr Wells has achieved the most brilliant results [mostly in ovariotomy] by taking care that there shall be few deleterious germs present at his operations. Mr Hutchinson has seemed to me to be as successful as Mr Lister with compound fractures by taking care to prevent the multiplication of germs by the application of cold. Mr Maunder and others, in their subcutaneous section, by which the entrance of germs *in a dangerous dose* is almost impossible, have attained extraordinary success.[60]

This very knowledgeable writer went on to complicate matters further by explaining (correctly) that what matters is the relation between the nature and volume of germs present and the total resistance of the organism — a point that Lister had not originally understood. Because of this, limiting the dose of germs may often be all that is required. But because the dose could not be measured, 'partial antiseptic practice is liable after periods of success to have sudden runs of disaster'.

The view that antiseptic surgery was only one among many changes that were reducing the death rate in surgical operations was founded on accurate observation. There were by the mid-1870s, undoubtedly, many Listerians, many partial Listerians, and many anti-Listerians, and, although the results of the antiseptic surgeons were on the whole probably the best, some at least of their opponents, as Godlee concedes, 'could show very excellent results indeed'.[61] There were cases where a surgeon achieved a high rate of success apparently because of his own individual attention to cleanliness, but more often the general surroundings in which the surgeon operated had also to be taken into account. These surroundings were changing. The point had sunk in at last that dirt and overcrowding bred disease. Even two people as dissimilar as the conservative Robert Barnes and the pioneering Spencer Wells could agree about this. The problem of pyaemia, wrote Barnes, is one of 'the convection of poison'. Once begun, pyaemia is spread 'in the articles of dress, the hospital appliances, the nurses, the students, and the surgeon himself'[62] Only a few months later Spencer Wells wrote of pyaemia that 'it is only in crowded hospitals that I have ever seen the disease'. It could be controlled or prevented, he wrote.

> by very great care in the treatment of wounds, by maintaining the wound in a state of perfect rest, by maintaining the most scrupulous cleanliness, by avoiding anything that can possibly injure the patient, locally or generally. . .

And he emphasised the point that because it was known that what patients needed was 'protection from contagion and infection', surgeons were no longer entitled to regard the outcome of operations as an act of God.

> People are apt to say, 'Oh, it does not matter. You do an operation, you cannot tell whether the patient is going to get well or not. You may do a slight operation and the patient will die, you may do a serious operation and he will get well, and you do not know why it is so.'[63]

But, said Spencer Wells, if a patient dies after a slight operation, 'the most rigid self-examination should be made by the surgeon'. It is a striking fact that this had to be said as late as 1874.

This general raising of standards was in part, no doubt, a response to Lister's work. But it was also in part a result of the hospitalism controversy. 'The fiery cross of hygiene', wrote one disgusted doctor in 1872, 'is now going through the land'.[64] It was none too soon. The improvement of hospitals that began, or is said to have begun, in the late eighteenth century does not seem to have achieved very much by the 1860s or even the 1870s. It is not easy to imagine what these mid-Victorian hospitals were like. They were dreadful places, even with chloroform. As Sir Eric Erichsen described them in the mid-1870s, they were:

> simply big houses, with basements containing kitchens, lavatories, cellars, and the ordinary offices of a large establishment, with an operating-theatre and dead-house more or less closely connected with the main building, with every floor filled with sick and wounded people; on the ground floor, accidents and operating cases; on the first floor, probably medical patients; above, chronic, surgical and medical cases. Who can wonder at the development of pyaemia below, and of erysipelas above? Who would live in an ordinary house thus filled? Who would expect to preserve his health if he ventured to inhabit it?[65]

The smell alone was appalling. When an empyema, containing very fetid pus, was opened in a ward in the large hospital at Netley, the smell, according to Simpson, 'was ere long felt and complained of in rooms or wards up to 500 feet distant on one side'.[66] As late as 1878 it was said that most of the surgeon's daily work 'is done in an atmosphere of foul emanations'; and, the author added, 'he is in almost constant contact with pus and septic products'.[67] For these and other reasons the hospitals were often full of flies. A surgeon in Glasgow during the hot summer of 1868 resorted to vaporising carbolic acid over a gas jet in order to get rid of the flies, 'so numerous and so annoying were they in wards not thus fumigated'. But during the 1870s the fiery cross made converts everywhere. Instead of being dark, smelly, dirty and overcrowded, hospitals began to be reasonably airy, reasonably clean, and reasonably spacious. The essential steps were to reduce the number of beds in a ward, perhaps by one-third, and to ensure a circulation of fresh air through the ward. The latter required that wards be reconstructed or new hospitals built. Before 1870 the wards were usually square, with one window, one fireplace, and one door leading into the passage. The window, open in summer, provided little draught, and in winter it was kept closed because of the cold. Another form of construction provided a long room with windows at both ends only. In this case, when both windows were open there was a good draught, but, it was lamented, 'the emanations from the patients to windward must pass over those to leeward'. What are now regarded as typical Victorian wards were all built in the last two or three decades of the nineteenth century. Another alteration that had to be made in the case of numerous hospitals was the provision of an adequate supply of clean water and observance of the ordinary habits of personal cleanliness. Nursing was also improved, although the targets set were not very high. In 1869, when St George's was 'taking steps to remodel its nursing establishment on a satisfactory basis', the aim was to have 331 beds and 55 nurses who, with bed, board and lodging ('no scrubbing required') were to receive from £18 to £20 per annum. Yet the changes brought about were, in aggregate, important and extensive. In 1875 the *Lancet* felt able to claim that 'in matters of hygiene no precaution is now too trivial'.[68] And the credit must go, in no small measure, to Simpson. Once again the world owed a debt of gratitude to the extraordinary energy and incessant action of this remarkable man. His analysis of the hospital problem, and his suggestions for putting things right, were hopelessly defective. And yet, although he stated the problem wrongly and proposed an impossible solution, he compelled acceptance of the idea that hospitals should and could be improved. His initiative and institution in this field, supported but corrected by Syme, Erichsen, and many others, saved countless lives. It changed the conditons in which surgeons worked. But for this reason it became virtually impossible to decide how far the better results of the later 1870s were due to the methods that many surgeons now employed, because they were being employed in healthier surroundings. Thus when Newcastle Infirmary announced in 1878 that a death rate in major amputations of 50 per cent had fallen after the introduction of antiseptic measures 'invariably and rigorously carried out, to a mere twelve per cent', it had to be added that 'other important sanitary improvements'[69] had been introduced at the same time; and which of all these changes reduced the death rate immediately became open to argument.

Thus antiseptic surgery was brought into use along with more or less antiseptic hospitals. Of course the better surgical technique and the more hygienic hospital surroundings reinforced one another. But contemporaries had some doubts. Spencer Wells, for example, who in the 1870s was probably the most distinguished pioneer in surgery after Lister himself, and who was always a fair and intelligent commentator, was concerned lest too much be expected of antiseptic techniques. Undue faith in the system, he wrote, 'may lead to rash practice and the attempt to do things which had better be left alone'. It was easy, he thought, to trust too far.

> I have more than once said, 'This sponge had better be burned', and the reply has been, 'Put it in one-to-twenty'. Only two days ago one of the most distinguished of the rising surgeons of the day told me that he had gone straight from a post-mortem examination to operate for strangulated hernia, quite confident that the spray and washing the hands with carbolised water would make him safe.

Spencer Wells also believed, like many others, that comfort and clean air mattered more than carbolic acid.

> For my part I would rather operate in a clean, quiet, well-warmed and well-ventilated building, be it large or small, without any antiseptic precautions, than run the risk of trusting to the neutralising or destructive power of chlorine or iodine, sulphur or tar, borax or the permanganates, salicylic or any other acid, in a place tainted by the presence of sewer-gas, or the seeds of some infections or contagious disease.[70]

Some even argued that if surgery was performed in antiseptic surroundings there was no need, or no great need, for it to be antiseptic in itself. This was put forward by the *Lancet*, for example, in 1879. If a 'pestilential atmosphere' exists, then Listerism is best. But the task of surgery is to establish the most favourable possible surroundings in which to operate, not to devise means which enable operations to be performed in dangerous surroundings. Antiseptic surgery is well enough, but what is of overriding importance is 'the antisepsis of cleanliness'.

> If special chemical agents [sic] are to be trusted to, and the established precautions of hygiene ignored, evil will sooner or later overtake us. Without these, these are unsafe; with these, they are, it is contended, unnecessary.[71]

There was some truth in this, except that by 1879 no responsible person proposed to ignore 'the established precautions of hygiene'. The quotation, however, illustrates a willingness, even an eagerness to do without antiseptic surgery if at all possible; and this eagerness was quite widespread. Probably one of its chief foundations was aversion to the complexity of Lister's technique. The best results, it was often said, were achieved by the simplest means. Others wanted, and used, a 'modified Listerism' along with good hygiene. Not a few considered that Lister 'had mixed up with his methods many details which were very repulsive to surgeons', or found 'the method . . . repellent, especially the operating with a cloud of spray on one's hands, and often in one's eyes'.[72]

In spite of all the objections, antiseptic surgery according to Lister gained a lot of ground during the 1870s. In Germany the antiseptic method was very widely accepted by 1875; Lister's tour through Germany in the summer of that year assumed, it was said, 'the character of a triumphal march'.[73] He returned to address the BMA at Edinburgh two months later, and

> impressed many steady-going practitioners by his bold and brilliant demonstrations of his method of dressing [sic]. By the exhibition of cases . . . and by appeals to startling operations performed in the fullest confidence of their ultimate success, Mr Lister in a few days gained more converts to the faith of his doctrines than many long years of teaching, writing and beseeching have been able to secure. It was no secret that many who went to scoff came away convinced. . . The system has grown and spread, and under its protection timid surgeons have shown a boldness which the bravest a few years ago scarcely dreamed of. . . In a word, Listerianism has been accepted by a very large section of surgical practitioners as synonymous with scientific surgery.[74]

Nothing was so persuasive as seeing Lister at work. Most of those who visited his wards in Edinburgh were, as one of them expressed it, 'driven to belief'.

There were many surgeons, however, mostly in London, who operated almost as if Lister had never written; who gave or believed they gave his methods a more or less prolonged trial and then, 'for weariness of the details, or dislike of the mechanical processes needed, and especially the disagreeableness of the spray during operations',[75] rejected them; or, at best, made free use of antiseptics while maintaining that 'the treatment should be carried out on a more simple plan, without that elaborate attention to detail which Mr Lister has thought necessary'.[76] At the end of 1875 the *Lancet* reckoned that in London 'it would be difficult to name more than one or two who are thorough-going believers in the theory, and there are scarcely more who strictly and fully carry out the practice'.[77]

There are several reasons why active opposition or a passive refusal to be interested were so strong in London. For one thing, London was the great rival of Edinburgh in particular and of Scotland in general as a scene of medical advance. For a hundred years an enormous number of significant medical discoveries had been made in Scotland, and the history of medicine in these years is astonishingly full of Scottish names. Also, a very high proportion of the medical men who staffed the expanding medical services in England during this period came from Scotland. The North of England and the rapidly growing Midlands were especially full of Scottish graduates, many of whom had come under Lister's influence either at Edinburgh or at Glasgow. But London kept itself aloof from this invasion. Few Scottish graduates obtained posts in London hospitals, and because the population growth of the metropolis was slower than that of many of the new industrial areas, promotion in the London hospitals was likewise slower and the older men retained control. They were almost all hostile to antiseptic surgery. Another innovation from north of the border was more than they could tolerate. Moreover, many of them subscribed to the view that an 'adequate improvement' in sanitary arrangements could achieve what was wanted, and this adequate improvement was possible in London because London tended to have more money than elsewhere. Callender, for example, worked in what a critic called 'the richest hospital in the world',[78] while Spencer Wells's hospital was 'like a private house'.[79] Given superior general conditions, inferior techniques might produce results not much less good than those of Lister.

Lister moved from Edinburgh to London in 1877 very largely, it would seem, because he thought this the only way in which he could finally persuade the London surgeons to adopt the antiseptic treatment. For he had learned to doubt whether much could be achieved by written explanation. 'It seems a difficult thing for me to write the English language so as to make my meaning intelligible. I find the opinion still often attributed to me that carbolic acid stops suppuration by some sort of specific agency.'[80] He came increasingly to rely on the younger men, whom he had taught personally, spreading the doctrine. He was 'the master' and they were 'the disciples'. It was in these apocalyptic terms that scientific surgery gained ground. And this conception of progress, that it depended upon a revelation understood only by the elect, was strengthened by the discovery that antiseptic surgery not only made safer what had been done before, but that it made possible many operations which before had never even been attempted. No man before Lister 'had laid open joints, clamped and cured fractured bones, drained the huge tuberculous abscesses which were then so common and so uniformly fatal in spinal disease, induced thrombosis in varicose veins or removed cancer, widely and radically, with all its lymphatic glands'.[81] The story often been told how in London in October 1877 Lister performed an 'open operation' on a broken kneecap by wiring the two fragments together, and how a prominent London surgeon said, or is supposed to have said, 'Now when this poor fellow dies, it is proper that someone should proceed against that man for malpractice'. Pre-Listerian surgeons — that is to say, the great majority of surgeons of Lister's age, or up to ten years younger — could not credit that operations of this kind were now possible. As far as they were concerned, they were not possible. And thus they were left behind in the progress of surgery. Lister 'felt it very necessary that the new operations should be undertaken only by those who had perfected themselves in the use of safeguards now available — by himself, that is to say, and by those who had been trained under his eye'.[82] His techniques, he thought, were the only passport into the greatly extended world of modern surgery. Those without this qualification were not welcome, and thus the division between the new surgeons and the old became more absolute. Distinguished men who did not accept the antiseptic technique found themselves excluded from, or at least found it more difficult to enter, the new realms of surgery. The threat to them — the proposal that Lister seemed to be making, so to speak — was that they would cease to be fully qualified members of the profession, that they would be transformed from men of experience into beginners. Hence arose the strength of their opposition, its persistence, its irrationality, its sound and fury, and its elements of common sense.

By the mid-and late 1870s uncertainty and consequent uneasiness were widespread. There was 'an uncomfortable feeling', as the *Lancet* put it, that the antiseptic method 'must somehow be brought in'.[83] But uncomfortable feelings and vague language were not going to solve the problem. Indeed, it seemed at this stage perfectly possible, even likely, that antiseptic surgery would fall back, so great was the emphasis on healthier hospital surroundings and so many were those surgeons who used and were satisfied with a modified antiseptic method.

There were two possible ways of resolving the difficulty. One was for some trial of Lister's method to be made which would conclusively demonstrate its superiority over any other method. Some asked why statistics were not assembled which would prove the point. Lister was repeatedly accused of suppressing statistics, or of being unable to produce statistics which would support his claims. But the difficulty is very real in surgical statistics that the cases compared are not really comparable, and that results said to be the same are not really so. Lister disliked and distrusted statistics (perhaps Simpson's misuse of them confirmed his worst suspicions) and in all his years of research and practice Lister himself published very few statistics. But after many years of silent resistance he allowed one of his house-surgeons, Watson Cheyne, to compile some on his behalf. These were published in 1879, and they helped in the final triumph of antiseptic surgery; but by that time many other arguments were equally persuasive. Others wanted some overt and planned comparison to be made. Holmes suggested in 1877 that Lister should continue his antiseptic work at King's College while Wood followed his own methods in the same hospital and the results be published and compared year by year. A year later it was proposed that 'if the London surgeons must have a rough and striking test' ten psoas abscesses should be opened by 'the champion of their choice' and another ten by Lister, the results to be published and compared; a sort of medieval knights' combat. To all such proposals there were obvious objections, but one in particular which Lister repeated several times. When you can open a healthy joint, he said, keep it open, and put in and frequently replace a drainage tube without causing any inflammatory disturbance whatever, you have 'a kind of fact of a new order, showing that we have a new principle at work'.[84] And this was indeed the fundamental and inescapable point. The antiseptic system depended on a theory. If the theory was right, the antiseptic system or something very like it had to be accepted. If the theory was wrong, then the problem had to be settled by purely empirical means, by simple trial and error. No doubt many adopted the practice, more or less, who ignored or denied the theory. But this was apt to have unfortunate results because, as Lister often said, those who did not have a firm belief in the theory could see no reason for extreme and unremitting care in practice; and so accidents occurred. What was needed for the final triumph of antiseptic surgery was acceptance of the theory that lay behind Lister's work. Gradually this came to be realised. As the 1870s wore on attention became focused increasingly not on Lister's practice but on what had been his point of departure: the germ theory of disease.

Lister's version of the germ theory concentrated on two items. First, germs are the cause of decomposition in wounds; second, germs are everywhere. Both these propositions were denied. For example, at the BMA meeting at Leeds in 1869 Professor Bennett of Edinburgh had only contempt for the daft idea that 'organic germs' might be the vehicle of contagion, for, as the *Lancet* put it, 'he had hunted these mythical germs for years with a fiftieth of an inch object glass, and had never caught them'.[85] A few months later Campbell Black in Glasgow wrote to say that 'it has never yet been proved that suppuration is due to sporules . . . their existence in the atmosphere is problematical . . . the germ theory of disease and contagion, of Lemaire and others, is untenable'. He added that 'this carbolic acid fuss' is 'frivolous and unscientific'.[86] Notions of the ubiquity of germs were equally roughly handled. James Morton, Professor of Materia Medica at Anderson's University in Glasgow claimed in 1870 that Pasteur's theory 'has not been satisfactorily established'. That the air is full of harmful germs, he said, is an ingenious idea.

> The simplicity of the supposition is quite enchanting; but . . . it is a pure assumption, and the probabilities are entirely against its truth. . . It is a fearful idea — fortunately, for thousands, a baseless theory — that there are formations in nature, and actually floating in the air, which are constantly in readiness to aid the grim king in his onslaughts upon frail humanity. Our human nature shudders at the thought.[87]

Some years later the *Lancet* was equally sceptical about what it called 'the panspermic hypothesis'. 'Mr Lister tells us that the air is, as it were, darkened with disease-producing germs.' But if this was so, the argument went, all earlier successes of surgery 'must be looked upon as inexplicable phenomena'.[88]

Long argument raged over these and related questions. In the 1850s and 1860s, the word germ was used not necessarily to mean the sporule of a fungus or any kind of bacteria but whatever was the origin or first cause of an illness. By 1870, however, the argument about germs was mainly about 'ovular germs' or what we would call bacteria. It is true that in the mid-1870s there was support for a time for the idea that putrefaction was caused not by germs but by 'atmospheric particles' or by a 'chemical ferment' destitute of vitality, yet endowed with a power of self-multiplication equal to that of the organism associated with it. This idea, as Lister said, was unsupported by scientific evidence, but, if accepted, required its adherents to follow the antiseptic system just as much as did the germ theory itself. On the other hand, some took the view that germs, if they were indeed the cause of disease, could not possibly be airborne, and that a belief in germs therefore 'involves the absolutely unreserved acceptance of the doctrine of spontaneous generation'.[89]

The debate of the 1870s was carried on principally by John Tyndall, Henry Charlton Bastian, and Burdon Sanderson. Tyndall, one of the best-known physicists of the day, was an early and firm supporter of the germ theory of disease. In 1876 and 1877 he published two very distinguished papers on the subject of airborne germs. His first contribution was to demonstrate not simply the existence but in an approximate fashion the amount of floating dust in the air. This he did by means of a concentrated beam of light, in which the floating dust became visible; and then, giving the dust time to settle, he showed that the beam of light was no longer defined and visible to the naked eye in the absence of the motes of dust. In another experiment all the dust in a flask was drawn into the electric field of an incandescent wire and destroyed, and the air became clear and 'invisible'. Moreover, he showed that sterilised putrescible solutions could be exposed to dust-free air without undergoing decomposition; but that these same solutions exposed to ordinary optically impure air would at once begin to grow moulds and bacteria. In short, 'the atmosphere is charged with a fine dust clearly of an organic nature, since it is destroyed by a red heat'.[90] In his second paper Tyndall demonstrated that bacteria pass through phases, in one state being destructible in five minutes by exposure to a temperature of 100°C, but in the other, which he considered as the germ state of the bacterium, being thermo-resistant to an extreme degree. A master of experiment, Tyndall did as much as Pasteur to render the doctrine of spontaneous generation incredible. His influence was very great, and some public experiments which he carried out in 1877 in order to demonstrate the germ theory 'crowded the lecture theatre of the Royal Institute to the roof'.[91]

Opposition to these ideas was led by Dr Henry Charlton Bastian, Professor of Pathology and Physician to University College Hospital. Bastian was an exponent of the idea, as it was expressed in 1870, that 'baceteria, vibrios and various simple fungi may develop when their chemical elements are brought into relation under otherwise favourable circumstances of light, heat and moisture'.[92] In trying to establish a chemical basis for the origin of life it may be said that Bastian was ahead of his time. It may also be said that the arguments he marshalled against the germ theory were not inconsiderable. He entered the controversy in 1872 with the publication of a very large volume entitled *The Beginnings of Life,* and in 1875, in one of the longest papers ever published in a single issue of the *Lancet,* he stated his case as follows.[93]

Proof that contagia are low organisms or living units which multiply destructively within the body is 'altogether wanting'; the more likely explanation of diseases like pyaemia is

> that contagious particles, whether composed of living or not-living organic materials, may initiate changes in the tissues and fluids with which they come into contact, which changes may be exaggerated as they spread, so as at last to implicate the blood.
> the blood.

Admittedly, bacteria are sometimes met with in diseased fluids and tissues; but far from these being the cause of disease they 'are for the most part actual pathological products, engendered within the body, or are descendents of organisms owing such an origin'. The grounds for this belief were —

1. the 'alleged causes of diseases' may be injected into the bloodstream of animals without ill effect;
2. 'even in healthy persons [bacteria] may be found in myriads'; for example, in the air-passages and the alimentary tract;
3. that there are distinct species of bacteria is no answer. Even Lister had admitted that the same bacterium may under ordinary circumstances be comparatively harmless but at other times 'generate products poisonous to the human economy' .
4. 'fresh and actively contagious menstrua' can survive treatment (such as exposure to boiling alcohol) generally recognised to be totally destructive to all forms of living matter. It is an unnecessary hypothesis to suppose, as some do, that bacteria possess 'a wonderful property of passing into a state of persistent inactivity or latent vitality' which enables them to resist destruction;
5. bacteria are found most abundantly in connection with dying tissue elements; it cannot be shown that they attack healthy tissue;
6. although absent from the blood of healthy individuals during life, human blood shortly after death may be found to be 'swarming with these organisms in every stage of growth'.

Lister, said Bastian, might for all practical purposes be right. But the simplest deduction consistent with the evidence was that disease and inflammation are the consequences of a chemical action initiated by a living organism *or* by a tissue element *or* of lifeless organic matter *or* 'by some mere physico-chemical influence'.

Bastian supported these arguments with experiments that showed, or were thought to show, that Pasteur was wrong. Bastian agreed with Pasteur that some infusions having a neutral or slightly alkaline reaction, would, after boiling and in suitably protected conditions, decay; but Bastian claimed that in addition some infusions having an acid reaction would, similarly treated, 'ferment and swarm with bacteria'. Argument on this point reached such a pitch that in 1877 Pasteur himself intervened. He pointed out that 15 years earlier he had noted 'that the sterilisation of organic liquids, when they are neutral or slightly alkaline, requires a temperature of higher than 100 °C' to prevent decomposition. Dr Bastian, however, had been content to heat 'his urine' and 'his potash' only to 100°C. Mixing them to obtain neutrality, he then found that they contained bacteria. This, said Pasteur, was inevitable. Thousands of liquids would behave similarly.[94]

Bastian and his supporters were unconvinced. Whatever Pasteur said, large number of people who tried to repeat his experiments found that boiled infusions, acid, alkaline or neutral, fermented when given subsequent protection from the atmosphere. And even when they did not, it was possible to fall back upon the argument that sterilised fluids remained sterile 'because the process of boiling kills all the living germs they may have contained, and at the same time impairs the virtues of the dissolved organic matter'.[95]

The trouble was, of course, that so many experiments did not prove what they were said to prove. Burdon Sanderson, who seems to have been the most perceptive and level-headed British pathologist of the day, remarked more than once that there were too many 'theories and general speculations of all kinds' and not enough facts. But, he said, there were a few facts 'confirmed by the most competent persons both in England and Germany'. These were:

1. organisms found in morbid tissue could be injected into animals without result;
2. bacteria could not be found in many patients suffering from fever;

on the other hand

3. 'in all destructive inflammations . . . bacteria are certainly present in the liquids of the destructively inflamed part';
4. all destructive inflammations are spreading inflammations, and Recklinghausen in Strasbourg had shown that in spreading erysipelas bacteria were to be found in the lymphatic spaces near the skin 'not in the advanced stage of the process, but at . . . the edge of extending inflammation'.

He concluded that there was a connection between bacteria and disease such that Bastian's position was 'an extremely difficult one'. Nevertheless, he said, if the question, 'Do you believe in the germ theory?' were put to the leading pathologists of the day, 'all of these eminent men would shrug their shoulders'.[96]

Amid such confusion of expert opinion it was inevitable that non-experts clung to some simple explanation. And that simple explanation was some variant of the idea of spontaneous generation, or what the *Lancet* called 'occult atmospheric influences tending to the production of erysipelas and pyaemia'.[97] When in 1874 the hospitalism debate seemed to be over, Sir John Eric Erichsen, senior surgeon at University College Hospital and a person of much influence, undertook to show that much mortality in hospitals was the result of 'a general morbid condition of the atmosphere productive of disease'. It was, he said, 'undoubted' that 'the septic poison which . . . impregnates a wound . . . is capable of transmission through the medium of the atmosphere'. Trouble arose, he explained, when 'morbid emanations' from suppurating wounds 'are developed too rapidly or too abundantly', causing the air to become 'overcharged with septic matters. . . At a certain point of impurity erysipelas and hospital gangrene appear.' The conclusion was, that Lister's insistence on cleanliness left nothing to be desired, whatever the theory might be. Erichsen's series of articles, four in all, shows him to have been a well-informed, intelligent, not unduly prejudiced and progressive surgeon. It is true that he believed that 'practical surgery has nearly, if not quite, attained finality'. But he also thought that the death rate in hospitals, especially after amputations, was excessive, and that it was 'dependent on determinable and removable causes, and might therefore be reduced, if not entirely abolished'; he understood what was being done in ovariotomy by Keith and Spencer Wells; he realised the disastrous consequences that might come from dirty sponges and dirty dressings; he considered that 'dissecting students' were 'by no means an uncommon cause of infection'; he thought that Simpson's figures on hospitalism proved nothing but that the repeated occurrence of hospital gangrene in a hospital 'would undoubtedly be discreditable to those who had the management of its sanitary arrangements'; and he even found it probable 'that there are different forms of septic disease'.[98] Erichsen was an enlightened surgeon. But, like many far less enlightened than himself, he saw no reason for going as far as Lister did.

Towards the end of the 1870s the evidence that Pasteur was right and that his opponents were wrong began to be irresistible. Most generally, men learned to distinguish between experiments that proved what they were said to prove and those that did not. Within the field of medical science, further research extended knowledge of the variety of organisms that might have to be considered: granules, micrococci, microzymes, 'mere granules passing as micrococci', moving organisms, still organisms, small micrococci, active moving granules, dumbbells, beads. The list began to seem endless. Against this, evidence accumulated that although the atmosphere might be full of germs of one sort or another, the proportion of morbific germs present might often be quite small. This explained the fact that surgery before Lister had not been a total failure. Wounds exposed to the atmosphere might heal quite satisfactorily; it depended on the nature and number of germs present. This fact compelled Lister to make a concession that greatly strengthened his case. He had come to realise, a few years before 1879, that there is some unexplained peculiarity in living tissue 'as distinguished from ordinary matter, that acts antiseptically, as we may say — prevents the development of septic organisms, on the same sort of principle, probably, as a healthy living plant resists parasitic fungi'.[99] Moreover, he had shown in the 1870s by means of an elaborate series of experiments that the likelihood of a putrescible fluid becoming infected by micro-organisms from without depended on the concentration of the poison. These discoveries weakened the case for what many regarded as Lister's excessive antiseptic precautions but put the principle of antisepsis on a sounder footing. Then in 1883 Metchnikoff announced his discovery of phagocytosis, that is, of the process whereby defending living cells, or phagocytes, are capable of absorbing and digesting invading micro-organisms. In this process, much turns on the numbers of germs involved; a few can be dealt with; large numbers overwhelm the defensive system. This discovery greatly strengthened the argument that living tissues should not be subjected to antiseptic washing or spraying because this damaged them (and thus weakened their powers of resistance) possibly as much as the washing or spraying killed the germs. Coupling this realisation with the knowledge that, in normal circumstances, the number of pathogenic organisms in the air was often not significantly large, surgeons came to see that the air was not, after all, the principal source of wound infection. The most important vehicles of danger were the patient's skin, the surgeon's hands, sponges, instruments, bandages, and particulate dirt of all kinds. The attempt to create an antiseptic atmosphere was therefore not so important after all. At the International Medical Congress in Berlin in 1890, Lister said,

> As regards the spray, I feel ashamed that I should ever have recommended it for the purpose of destroying the microbes in the air. If we watch the formation of the spray and observe how its narrow initial cone expands as it advances, with fresh portions of air continually drawn into its vortex, we see that many of the microbes in it, having only just come under its influence, cannot possibly have been deprived of their vitality. Yet there was a time when I assumed that such was the case. . .[100]

Lister's abandonment of the spray, ten years after it had been abandoned by even his most devoted admirers in Germany, came much too late to affect the general outcome: antiseptic surgery had been almost completely accepted in Britain long before 1890. It is of course impossible to give a precise date for Lister's triumph. But a paper published by Watson Cheyne in May 1879, and a debate on antiseptic surgery held by the South London Branch of the BMA in December of the same year clearly reduced Lister's opponents to a small and rapidly dwindling minority.

Watson Cheyne, who was described towards the end of his career as a true man of science and a better operator than Lister, had graduated at Edinburgh in 1875 and became Lister's house-surgeon in 1877. His paper[101] bore a startling title: *The Occurrence of Organisms under Antiseptic Dressings*. It sounded like a set-back for Lister, and his enemies must have read it with eagerness. The idea was not new. Several German investigators had reported finding organisms in antiseptically treated wounds. Watson Cheyne therefore examined the discharges from wounds. Because an observer using a microscope could not be sure of finding micrococci even when present in considerable numbers, Watson Cheyne inoculated prepared infusions with a drop of discharge. He found that in cases treated by Lister the inoculated fluid either remained clear or became turbid from the development of micrococci. In cases not treated in a thoroughly antiseptic manner, bacilli as well as micrococci grew in the infusions. He pointed out that micrococci were round cells which grew from pairs into chains or groups, and that there was no evidence that they developed from or into rod-shaped bacteria, as was sometimes stated. He further noted that infusions containing bacilli changed radically, whereas those containing only micrococci changed much less. Moreover, he found that fluids containing bacilli killed rabbits when injected into the jugular vein, those containing only micrococci did not.

Watson Cheyne then asked the crucial question, Why do micrococci flourish under antiseptic dressings, whereas bacilli do not? This must be the result, he reasoned, either of spontaneous generation; or because they are in any case present in the blood; or because they pass through the dressing. The first of these explanations he rejected because the infusions, when protected from the atmosphere and not inoculated, did not putrefy. The second he rejected because he found that micrococci did not flourish in 'healthy' blood, and because previous experiments purporting to show that organs taken from newly-killed animals contained bacteria were radically defective; Watson Cheyne gave good reasons for believing that the germs which were observed had entered these organs *after* their removal from the body. (This was important because Lister, as he subsequently said, had never believed that bacteria existed in the organs of healthy animals, and 'when he first heard of observations to the contrary he was staggered, for they were opposed to the fundamental facts of antiseptic surgery'.[102] This left entry through the dressing as the sole possibility, and Watson Cheyne was able to show both that carbolic acid weakens rapidly through evaporation and mixing with body fluids, and that micrococci are less sensitive to carbolic acid than are bacilli. The practical conclusion was the discharge from the wound, especially if profuse, might be insufficiently diluted by the carbolic acid in even a good antiseptic dressing to prevent the appearance of micrococci. These, 'which abound far more than bacteria[103] do in the ward atmosphere, find this [discharge] a favourable medium for growth; as they grow they increase in vigour and are able to live in fluid containing a larger proportion of carbolic acid; and if time be given, they will ultimately reach the wound'. Other findings which Watson Cheyne listed were of a more general nature and of no less importance. He had proved *inter alia:*

> That micrococci are distinct from bacteria in their mode of growth, in their relation to reagents and carbolic acid, in their effects on fluids and on the living body, and by the fact that they have never

been observed to pass one into the other. That the ordinary forms of micrococci are harmless in the body, contrasting markedly with the bacteria, which are so harmful . . . Finally, that the entrance of bacteria through dressings is the result of carelessness, and their entrance from the body can happen only in the most grave disturbance of the vital functions.

This paper is of considerable importance for three distinct reasons. First, it shows a mastery of experimental method. Watson Cheyne was not content to say, as so many of his contemporaries were, that germs were not present if they could not be seen through a microscope; he thought about, and exposed the defects in, the experimental methods of others, even of Germans, and thus could reject erroneous conclusions; in his own investigation each result led him to ask another question, and to conduct another experiment. Experimental work of so high an order was conclusive to a degree uncommon in British medical science in the 1870s, and it was an example to others. Secondly, some of Watson Cheyne's conclusions were very important; they revealed more than once what Lister called, with reference to his own results, 'a kind of fact of a new order'. In particular, there was the operational distinction between bacilli and micrococci. The distinction itself was not new; Robert Koch had suggested that there might be many forms of micrococci and Lister himself in 1873 had provided 'distinct physiological proof of real differences among bacteria'[104] but Watson Cheyne spelt out the reasons that made the distinction a very important one. He also brought forward the novel and enormously significant fact that minute organisms were able, within limits, to adapt to their environment. Lastly, and in a way most important of all, Watson Cheyne's paper is the first contribution, certainly the first important contribution, made to the theory and practice of antiseptic surgery by anyone other than Lister. Hitherto, there had been many who agreed with  Lister, and many more who disagreed. But no one had said: Lister is right; but there are also the following points. This was support of a new kind. Lister expressed surprise at learning that any organisms could exist under an antiseptic dressing, but he accepted the findings without hesitation. No doubt he realised that in the person of Watson Cheyne a pupil had grown into a very powerful ally. But he may not have realised that the constructive exchange of ideas within antiseptic surgery enormously increased its resilience, adaptability, and strength, and transformed an outpost of ideas into a self-reinforcing citadel.

Seven months later the South London Branch of the BMA gave

Lister an opportunity to restate his case and to rebut twelve years of accumulated criticism. His performance on this occasion can only be described as superb.[105]

After three or four speakers had given their opinion, ranging from full acceptance of antiseptic surgery to the view that it was a good idea but not really necessary, Lister rose to address the meeting. He dealt first with the often-repeated charge that if antiseptic surgery could do all that he claimed, this should be provable by statistics. 'I have often been reproached', he said,

> for not having produced statistics, and it has been hinted, and the hint has been lately pretty strongly reproduced, that I have suppressed statistics because I had none which I should not be ashamed to produce. Sir, the truth is that life is short, and that when every day begins one has to consider what is the occupation which is most likely to be valuable, and feeling, as I do . . . I have felt that there was every day something both more congenial and, I hoped, more profitable to do, than to compile statistics. . .

Nevertheless, Lister went on, it was not the case that he had withheld statistics regarding hospital diseases.

> When I left Glasgow I published a statistical account with reference to these diseases, and showed, as far as I could judge, that there had come over my wards, which previously had been amongst the most unhealthy in the kingdom, a wonderful change, a surprising alteration since the introduction of the antiseptic treatment; while in other wards in the same hospital, the old conditions remained unchanged.

But more is asked for.

> It is not sufficient to say that I have had only one case of pyaemia in five years in a great hospital, with an average of sixty patients under my charge, but you want me to say I have had so many amputations with no pyaemia, so many excisions of the mamma with no pyaemia, and so forth. I confess I do not see the force of that argument, for if I could be supposed guilty of making the false statement of having only one case of pyaemia in five years with sixty beds under my charge, I should be equally capable of compiling a false table of statistics.

A very good sample of surgical statistics had recently been published by Mr Savory, Lister went on, relating to St Bartholomew's Hospital for the three years from 1876 to 1878. These results 'show a noble amount of surgical success, [which] not many years ago would have been considered almost incredible'. Three of the four surgeons concerned, however, used antiseptic methods, two of them in a thorough-going manner. In spite of this, Lister provided a long and very detailed comparison of these results with what he had achieved in Edinburgh from November 1871 to August 1877. In this period he had carried out 845 operations with a death rate of 4.4 per cent. Savory, he said, gave figures only for 'major operations', which is 'very vague and arbitrary'. Lister was willing to call 725 of his operations 'major', although 'I cannot help remembering how easy it would have been for me to manipulate these statistics a little, and to make the result look better'. However, in his 725 so-called 'major' operations 37 of the patients died, giving a death rate of 5.1 per cent, not much better than Savory's 5.8 per cent. But, said Lister, only 6 of his patients died from blood-poisoning, whereas the St Bartholomew's rate was almost double. Moreover, 'there is a very weighty saying attributed to Morgagni, to this effect, *Perpendendae non numerandae observationes*', or 'Cases should be pondered, not numbered'. Some operations — lithotomy, for example, or those in the mouth — cannot be rendered antiseptic. Removing these operations from the list left 553; and in these 553, two patients died.

Lister then turned to deal with the topic so often at the forefront of surgical discussion, major amputations. He referred to Simpson's figures, generally accepted, which gave a mortality rate for amputations in city hospitals for many years before 1870 of between 35 per cent and 45 per cent. From 1871 to 1877 he himself, he said, had carried out 80 major amputations, with a death rate of 11.25 per cent. He then took his audience through the details of these operations, to show how little importance could be attached to the figure of 11.25 per cent. The facts were as follows:

One patient was 'moribund on admission. I operated practically without any hope of saving the man.'

One was an operation 'of tremendous difficulty, and the patient sank as the immediate result of the operation'.

One case required two operations, which 'reduced that man so much that within twenty-four hours he was dead'.

Two other cases 'were in a state of collapse before the operation, and neither rallied'.

One case 'was in a state of collapse when he was admitted, and never rallied'.

One case (a malignant tumour of the arm) 'was doing perfectly well, but after some time the patient died of haemorrhage from another tumour in the femur, of the existence of which we were not aware'.

One case 'died from diphtheria. As far as the amputation was concerned, it was a case of recovery.'

I had eighteen amputations of the ankle, and of these one patient died, but that was a boy who three months after the operation, when the wound was almost absolutely healed, died of cerebral haemorrhage. With regard to the amputation this also was a case of recovery.

Then, Lister continued, there were those cases which used to be considered exceedingly dangerous because of the risk of pyaemia; cases of ununited fracture treated by cutting down on the seat of the fracture and removing the ends of the fragments.

We used to operate thus upon some of these cases in the upper limb, but in the lower we considered that the risk of pyaemia was so great as to prohibit the procedure. In the five and three-quarter years I have referred to I have operated eight times for ununited fracture of the thigh, nine times for ununited fracture of the leg, once for ununited fracture of the clavicle, four times for ununited fracture of the humerus, and five times for ununited fracture of the forearm — in all, twenty-six cases, and so far as I know all these patients are alive and well — not one of them died.

These figures were convincing enough; indeed, they formed in themselves an almost overwhelming case for antiseptic surgery. But Lister was far from finished. It remained the essence of his argument that statistics were subordinate to physiological and surgical understanding. What mattered, he insisted, was that very often his statistics demonstrated a new principle in surgery. This was the real force of his argument to which his opponents had no reply; and on this occasion he drove the point home with relentless iteration.

I may be wrong, but it seems to me that, if you were to open a healthy joint, keep the wound open and put a drainage-tube into it, and take that drainage-tube out every day and wash it, and put it in again, not using antiseptic means of some sort or other, you would infallibly have more or less of inflammatory disturbance, and it would be impossible to have the condition of things which we now look upon as normal — namely, no tenderness, no blush of redness, no puffiness, no uneasiness, not to mention no suppuration. As far as I am able to judge, this is a kind of face of a new order, showing that we have a new principle at work.

It is no good saying that 'the publication of isolated cases, however good, proves nothing'.

I say that one individual case, if it shows new pathological facts, is worth as much as a million. I have published, for instance, numerous cases to show that a great abscess connected with disease of the vertebrae may be opened by free incision, a drainage-tube introduced, strict antiseptic treatment being used, and that from that hour there is not another drop of pus. I believe this is a fact as new to pathology as it is beautiful in practice. Then I have pointed out again and again that you may have exposed in an open wound a blood-clot, no matter how large; and that this blood-clot may remain not only free from putrefaction, but indefinitely without suppuration, so that in the course of time, when you remove its upper surface, you find a scar beneath, without a drop of pus or a granulation having ever been formed. This again, as far as I am able to judge, is new in the history of surgery, and indicates that we have a new principle at work. Further, I have given evidence to show that dead tissue, if protected from putrefaction and also from the stimulation of antiseptic substances, may be absorbed in a way that I had never before supposed possible; that even a large piece of dead bone may have granulations grow over it; and these overlapping granulations may, as it were, eat it away till it is reduced to a very small size. That again, as far as I can judge, is an indication of a new principle.

Nor did Lister fail to remind his audience about the catgut ligature — 'how there is an absorption of dead tissue, and how living tissue comes to take its place. That, I say, is something quite new.'

Lister might have concluded his remarks at this point, having now spoken for about 80 minutes. But he wisely went on to make brief reference to the attitude of his critics, replying to them, as he usually did, more in sorrow than in anger. 'If these matters have not attracted attention', he said,

it cannot be because they are not worthy of it; I presume it is because I have not capacity to bring them before my professional brethren with sufficient force to impress them upon them. It is not, I say, that these things are unimportant; but they are not believed. With regard to the operation for transverse fracture of the patella, to which reference has been made, instead of its being thought probable that no harm would come of it, it was supposed to be a most dangerous operation, and hints were thrown out that if anything went wrong with the patient I ought to be brought up for manslaughter. With regard to abscesses, one of our best provincial surgeons was at King's College, and saw some of the cases there. He said, 'Do you mean to tell me that in the case of a great psoas abscess connected with disease of the vertebrae no pus is formed from the time you squeeze out the original contents?' He seemed to think that the thing was only made out a day or two before, instead of being a matter of practice for years past. Then as regards the organisation of the blood-clot. I know that this has been simply discredited, but I will not occupy the time of this great meeting by going into the evidence showing that this process really takes place. Nor will I dwell upon the absorption of dead bone, but I would like to say a word or two about the catgut ligature. It has been said, 'Oh, the organisation of the catgut ligature is all nonsense; the ligature is dissolved'. I confess I do not understand how it is that some gentlemen are disposed to believe the more unlikely thing rather than the natural and the probable one. Ask any chemist, is it a probable thing that a piece of catgut would be dissolved, even if put into pure water, unless it putrefied? . . . the substance of the catgut is an insoluble substance. . . Let anyone try the experiment; let him put the catgut, as I have done, into putrid serum for any length of time − it will not be dissolved, however long it is there. Then let him put it into non-putrid serum . . . and he will find that the catgut will not be dissolved. It is not a matter of dissolution, it is a matter of absorption by the living tissues. . . I am sometimes ashamed for my own professional brethren and their scientific credit.

Finally, Lister apologised to his audience for having detained them so long, and thanked them for having listened to him so patiently. In such a gathering of medical men, he said, he could not refrain from speaking warmly on a matter so near to his heart.

> I have been charged with enthusiasm, but I regard enthusiasm with reference to the avoidance of death, pain, and calamity to our fellow-creatures as a thing not at all to be ashamed of; for I feel this to be a matter of which I may say in the words of Horace —
> 'Aeque pauperibus prodest, locuphitibus aeque,
> Aeque neglectum pueris senibusque nocebit.'

In some ways Lister was not a good public speaker. He was always earnest, never amusing, and frequently took far more time than was allotted to him. These characteristics were no help in overcoming incredulity or hostility. But by 1879 most surgeons were at least half converted, and everyone had to take Lister's ideas seriously. In these circumstances he was enormously impressive. There was never anything slipshod in his arguments any more than in his surgery, and he stated a position with care and the utmost accuracy. On this occasion his rehearsal of so many arguments, his piling of case upon case, fact upon fact, deduction upon deduction, was overwhelming. The meeting was adjourned for a fortnight, but in reality it was concluded. A week later the *Lancet* acknowledged that 'the testimony of men holding the highest positions in the profession is such as to render it impossible for us to entertain any doubt whatever regarding the very great advantage to be derived from a strict adherence to Mr Lister's system of dressing wounds'.[106]

Inevitably, criticism and opposition did not fade away overnight. The *Lancet* remained sceptical about the germ theory, in spite of Robert Koch's epoch-making *Aetiology of Traumatic Infective Diseases*, published in 1878, and soon to be followed by Alexander Ogston's conclusive demonstrations that micrococci produce inflammation and suppuration. Lawson Tait admitted the truth of the germ theory but said that antiseptic precautions, at least in ovariotomy, delayed healing and tended to cause constitutional disturbance.[107] Sir James Paget claimed that mortality in his operations had fallen from over 15 per cent in 1847–57 to 10 per cent in 1857–67 and to less than 5 per cent in 1867–77 and that this was not because of antiseptic practices but because bleeding, leeching and purging had been abandoned and sanitation improved. Lister, he said, had made an important contribution simply because he 'provoked others to scrupulous care in the treatment of their cases'.[108] But these were the views of a minority.

Before the end of 1897 the *Lancet*, which had for so long sat on the fence, declared in round terms that 'Listerism is destined to be the surgery of the future',[109] and referred a year later to Lister's papers on antisepsis as having 'made an epoch in surgery'.[110] Honours accumulated upon him, given not only by the Germans, who had long ago recognised the importance of his contribution, but by his own countrymen. At the end of 1880 the Royal Society awarded him the Royal Medal, and in 1885 he was offered, but felt obliged to decline, the Presidency of the Royal College of Surgeons. Only in France doubt continued, but in a way that may have moved even Lister to mirth. There were two opposite points of view. On the one hand, it was claimed that

> the so-called treatment of Lister is essentially French. The drain belongs to Chassaignac; Lemaire was the originator of carbolic acid applications; Boinet claims the merit of opening abscesses, and washing them out with antiseptics; and the search for immediate union belongs to the French school to which is also due the catgut ligature. The only thing original in the method is the spray, and that has been shown to be useless.[111]

On the other hand, according to another French surgeon writing at the same time, 'Listerism depuis quelques années, après avoir fait le tour du monde, envahit la France et y exerce les ravages d'un véritable épidémie antiseptique'.[112]

## Notes

1. Von Volkmann, quoted in H.C. Cameron, *Joseph Lister, the Friend of Man* (London, 1948), p. 134.
2. Cameron, *Joseph Lister, the Friend of Man*, pp.k, 5, 148.
3. Letter dated July 1864, quoted in Cameron, *Joseph Lister*, p. 69.
4. In 1871 Lister prefaced his address to the BMA by saying that the antiseptic treatment 'is calculated, I believe, to revolutionise every department of surgery'. G.T. Wrench, *Lord Lister, His Life and Work* (London, 1913), p. 245.
5. *Lancet*, vol. II, (24 August, 1867), p. 234.
6. *Lancet*, vol. II, (1870), p. 400.
7. Quoted in Godlee, *Lord Lister*, p. 211.
8. *Lancet*, vol. I, (2 January, 1869), p. 47 (Charing Cross Hospital).
9. *Lancet*, vol. II, (1867), p.95.
10. *Lancet*, vol. II, (5 December, 1868), p. 728.
11. Ibid.
12. Lemaire, de L'Acédie Phénique, (etc) (Paris, 1863; 2nd edn 1865).

13. *Lancet*, vol. II, (5 October, 1867), p. 444.

14. Ibid., (19 October), p. 502.

15. Ibid., (2 November), pp. 546 ff.

16. *Lancet*, (9 November, 1967), p. 595.

17. See *Edinburgh Monthly Journal of Medical Science*, vol. IX, (November 1848), pp. 329 ff.

18. *British Medical Journal*, vol. II, (1867), p. 282.

19. Quoted in Godlee, *Lord Lister*, p. 135.

20. *Lancet*, vol. II, (1869), p. 296.

21. Ibid., p. 332.

22. *Lancet*, vol. II, (1869), p. 432.

23. Ibid., p. 699.

24. J.Y. Simpson, *Puerperal*, Lecture Notes for 1840, Notebook No. 11, in the Royal College of Physicians, Edinburgh.

25. D. Zuck, 'Simpson as a Teacher — a Student's Notebook', in *British Journal of Anaesthesia*, (1976), 48, 1103.

26. *Monthly Journal of Medical Science*, vol. XI, (November 1850), pp. 414 ff.

27. Proceedings of the Medico-Chirurgical Society of Edinburgh, (16 April 1851), in *Monthly Journal of Medical Science,* vol. XIII (July 1851), pp. 70 ff.

28. See *Monthly Journal of Medical Science*, vol. XII, (June 1851), pp. 505 ff.

29. see ibid., vol. XIII, (July 1851), pp. 70 ff.

30. *Lancet*, vol. II, (1869), p. 451.

31. *Lancet*, vol. II, (1871), p. 550.

32. Ibid., p. 551.

33. Ibid.

34. *Lancet*, vol. I, (1 January, 1870), pp. 4 ff.

35. *Lancet,* vol. I (1870), pp. 4–5.

36. Ibid., (29 January, 1870), p. 175.

37. *Lancet*, vol. II, (1873), p. 185.

38. Ibid., (6 September), p. 353.

39. *Lancet*, vol. I, (3 January, 1874), p. 9.

40. The method was 'to bring the cases one by one into a room, where the students are comfortably seated . . . [to point out] their distinctive characters . . . having done this . . . the teacher proceeds to explain the principles of treatment, with his reasons for choosing the method preferred . . . *Lancet*, vol. II, (1864), p. 391.

41. *Lancet*, vol. II, (28 August, 1869),  p. 320.

42. Ibid., (18 September), p. 421.

43. *Lancet,*  vol. II, (1870), p. 287.

44. Godlee, *Lord Lister* p. 212.

45. *Lancet*, vol. I, (1870), p. 91.

46. *Lancet*, vol. I (1873), p. 729.

47. *Lancet*, vol. I, (1870), p. 317.

48. *Lancet*, vol. I, (1869), p. 380.

49. Ibid.

50. Quoted in Wrench, *Lord Lister, His Life and Work*, p. 262.

51. *Lancet*, vol. I, (1871), p. 45.

52. L. Tait, *Medico-chirurgical Transactions* (1880), p. 161.

53. *British Medical Journal*, vol. II, (1890), p. 732.

54. *Lancet*, vol. I, (1880), p. 666.

55. *British Medical Journal,* vol. I, (1899), p. 1561.

56. *Lancet,* vol. II, (28 August, 1869), p. 320.

57. *Lancet*, vol. I, (1879), p. 65.

58. Ibid.

59. Ibid.
60. *Lancet*, vol. I, (1878), p. 36.
61. Godlee, *Lord Lister*, p. 288.
62. *Lancet*, vol. I, (1874), p. 179.
63. Ibid., p. 411.
64. *Lancet*, vol. II, (1872), p. 122.
65. *Lancet*, vol. I, (1874), p. 223.
66. *Lancet*, vol. II, (20 November, 1869), p. 699.
67. *Lancet*, vol. II, (1878), p. 188.
68. *Lancet*, vol. II, (16 October, 1875), p. 565.
69. *Lancet*, vol. II, (16 August, 1879), p. 247.
70. *Lancet*, vol. I, (1978), p. 134.
71. *Lancet*, vol. II, (16 August 1879), p. 247.
72. *Lancet*, vol. II, (1875), p. 628.
73. *Lancet*, vol. I, (19 June, 1875), p. 868.
74. *Lancet*, vol. II, (16 August, 1879), p. 246.
75. *Lancet*, vol. II, (20 November, 1875), p. 743.
76. *Lancet*, vol. I, (1875), p. 692.
77. Ibid.
78. Quoted in Wrench, *Lord Lister, His Life and Work*, p. 266.
79. Ibid., p. 267.
80. Quoted in Comeron, *Joseph Lister, the Friend of Man*, p. 101.
81. Ibid., p. 92.
82. Ibid.
83. *Lancet*, vol. I, (1875), p. 692.
84. *Lancet*, vol. II, (6 December, 1879), p. 854.
85. *Lancet*, vol. II, (7 August, 1869), p. 201.
86. Ibid., p. 524.
87. *Lancet*, vol. I, (29 January, 1870), p. 155.
88. *Lancet*, vol. II, (23 October, 1875), p. 597.
89. *Lancet*, vol. II, (1870), p. 714.
90. Ibid., p. 923.
91. *Lancet*, vol. I, (1877), p. 145.
92. *Lancet*, vol. II, (1870), p. 923.
93. *Lancet*, vol. I, (1875), p. 501 ff.
94. *Lancet*, vol. I, (1877), p. 332.
95. Bastain in the *Lancet*, vol. I, (1867), p. 206.
96. *Lancet*, vol. I, (1875), p. 511.
97. *Lancet*, vol. II, (23, August, 1873), p. 272.
98. *Lancet*, vol. I, (1874), pp. 84, 124, 151 and 221 ff.
99. *Lancet*, vol. II, (1879), p. 457.
100. Quoted in Godlee, *Lord Lister*, p. 291.
101. *Lancet*, vol. I, (17 May, 1879), p. 703.
102. *Lancet*, vol. II, (1879), p. 704.
103. In this and the following passage Watson Cheyne uses the word bacteria to mean what we would call bacilli.
104. 'On the Germ Theory of Putrefaction and other Fermentative Changes', in *Nature,* Part XLV, vol. VIII, (10 July, 1873), p. 212.
105. There is a fairly full account in the *Lancet*, vol. II, (1879), pp. 850 ff.
106. *Lancet*, vol. II, (13 December, 1879), p. 882.
107. *Lancet*, vol. I, (1880), p. 250.
108. *Lancet*, vol. II, (1879), p. 923.

109. *Lancet*, vol. II, (1879), p. 915.
110. *Lancet*, vol. II, (1880), p. 984.
111. *Lancet*, vol. I, (1879), p. 575.
112. *Lancet*, vol. II, (1880), p. 984.

# 6   THE FIGHT FOR NEW IDEAS

It is beyond question that inhalation anaesthesia and antiseptic surgery were two of the greatest innovations ever made in medical theory or practice; the only other advances of comparable importance would be Harvey's discovery of the circulation of the blood, Jenner's introduction of vaccination, Pasteur's demonstrations of the nature of putrefaction and the process of active immunisation, and perhaps Fleming's discovery of penicillin. In spite of the profound and far-reaching consequences of what Simpson and Lister proposed, or perhaps because of them, their ideas were met in many professional quarters with indifference or opposition, and such attitudes continued for several years.

That new ideas in any sphere of life are often met with hostility is a well-known fact. Whatever is established is of proven usefulness, its limitations as well as its value are understood, it has the support of time, and perhaps also of famous and respected names; on the other hand, what is new is yet untried. Moreover, new devices or new technologies or even new designs are likely to require the users to learn and to adapt, and learning and adaptation are not agreeable to everyone, especially to those who are old enough to be set in their ways of thinking and doing. Even new ways of producing, unaltered, old goods or services may be unwelcome by causing or threatening to cause unemployment among producers. An innovation, even an apparently minor innovation, is likely to set going ripples or shock-waves of change through any kind of organisation, be it a family or a business enterprise or a profession or any other group.

There is nothing new in all this, certainly not in medicine. Harvey once said that no man over 40 was willing to adopt his doctrine of the circulation of the blood. What contemporaries found so hard to accept in Harvey's work was that his views ran counter to the Galenic tradition, a tradition that was supported, as Harvey himself said, 'by such a host of learned and distinguished men'. His teaching gravely disturbed the confidence and mental repose of others: 'by setting down the circulatory motion of the blood innumerable axioms of ancient writers were overturned; whence it comes that all the order of teaching is troubled'.[1] Over one hundred years later Jenner and his followers likewise met resistance. In part this sprang from religious prejudice,

which held that to be immunised against smallpox was to interfere with
the workings of divine providence, but most of it came from medical
men, among whom the most vocal were those whose incomes depended
on the specialised practice of inoculating with the actual smallpox
virus. Simpson knew about the reception that Jenner's discovery had received, and when opposition to his own ideas developed he wrote a forceful article pointing out that the objections to vaccination had been
crushed out of existence by accumulated facts, and predicting that 'a
sufficient body of accurate and well-ascertained facts' about anaesthesia
would likewise, in a short time, triumph over mere opinion and prejudice.
There were other instances of mistaken conservatism to which Simpson
could have appealed. The originator of the theory of percussion was
met, as he said he expected to be met, 'by envy, malice, hatred, detrac-
tion, and calumny', and his work was totally neglected in his own
lifetime. When the stethoscope began to come into use in the United
States, it was noted by Oliver Wendell Holmes that 'the old, hard-
working operatives' were less inclined to acknowledge its usefulness
than to 'observe and signalize all the errors and defects which happened
in its practical application'. The same human reaction among doctors
had occurred in respect of vaccination, almost as much attention being
paid to the fact that revaccination was necessary, and that serious
complications sometimes ensued, as to the enormous benefits that were
secured.[2]

But why are such reactions of resistance and opposition so common?
Do we have to attribute them simply to an inherent conservatism in
human nature, and leave it at that? Or is a large part played by mere
reluctance to think? Or is it less a matter of human nature than of
institutional arrangements? In any society, after all, and especially in
a technologically complex society, new ideas, although they may be
originated by individuals, are transmitted through institutional arrangements of one kind or another. But how wide-spreading are these
institutional arrangements? How do they work to facilitate or oppose?
How important are individuals in all this process, either the innovators
themselves or some of the resisters? How much can be explained by
current circumstances and how much depends on the past? To what
extent is doubt or even opposition justified? Are the arguments largely
technical, or do they spread into quite different fields from the one
primarily concerned? Is it simply a practical matter, or are points of
principle involved? Of course no general answer, covering all instances,
can be given to these questions. But the evidence of the preceding
chapters suggests that the processes of resistance and persuasion may be

very far from simple.

In the case of chloroform there were two, and in the case of antisepsis three, principal grounds of opposition. As regards chloroform, a good deal of resistance was based on the facts that incorrect or careless exhibition of the drug was easy and in the early years not uncommon, and that the results could be fatal. Unlike ether, chloroform was dangerous; and unlike any other drug in general use at that time, it could kill a patient in a few minutes, almost without warning. Simpson had, in fact, put into general circulation a first-class poison. To begin with, the dangers of chloroform anaesthesia were not generally understood and several patients, admittedly a very small proportion of those put under chloroform, lost their lives. But what is remarkable, and important, is that from the very start Simpson and Snow and one or two other pioneers of chloroform anaesthesia such as Syme and Protheroe Smith understood very well and stated very clearly how patients could be anaesthetised with safety. It has to be admitted that some intelligent and conscientious doctors may have found the experts' advice a little difficult to follow. The 'Scots rules' were a descriptive guide rather than a scientific formula and so could be misinterpreted; Snow, on the other hand, aimed for a quantitative and therefore 'objective' control of inhalation by means of the inhaler – but inhalers could be mishandled. Nevertheless, the administrator who took care to exhibit chloroform vapour diluted with air and who paid careful, not casual, attention to the patient's respiration could hardly go wrong. That enough was known about chloroform anaesthesia to make it safe from the beginning is proved by the fact that between 1847-60 Syme, Snow and Simpson anaethetised approximately 15,000 patients between them, and did not have a single fatality.[3] Most of the trouble arose from the profession's failure to understand and apply the technique as it was taught. Some, who lacked confidence, exhibited chloroform much diluted with air and induced only struggling and excitement. It is even possible that a few patients died in this way, for light anaesthesia can cause ventricular fibrillation of the heart with possibly fatal consequences. Others, bolder but careless, gave an over-dose, and either killed the patient at once or continued the chloroform in spite of stertorous or interrupted breathing. Others, again, exhibited chloroform that was impure or downright lethal. All such mistakes were a reflection on the ability of the medical profession to understand and follow sound professional advice. And this means that resistance to chloroform anaesthesia because it was dangerous amounted to a confession of incompetence by the doctors themselves.

The other major objection to chloroform anaesthesia, applying only in midwifery, was a miscellaneous assortment of medical, sociological, ethical and religious objections. Chloroform, it was maintained, weakened the action of the uterus and thus endangered mother and child by delaying birth; it was improper and unnatural, perhaps it was even wrong, that a woman should not be fully conscious during the birth of her child, and suffer accordingly; to reduce or eliminate her agonies, others said, was to thwart the Almighty. Only the first of these arguments was strictly medical; on the other hand, medical and ethical problems (in the widest sense) are frequently inseparable.

The very fact that this is such a hotch-potch of arguments arouses suspicion. Do they represent more than a medley of deep-seated Victorian male prejudices? To answer this question conclusively would require long and thorough investigation, but mere prejudice or preference is what it all looks like. The medical argument about delaying birth was wrong, unless the mother was narcotised to a quite unnecessary and possibly dangerous degree; and this argument soon ceased to be heard. The religious objections likewise did not last very long. When chloroform was first used in midwifery, then, as one doctor put it, 'many serious-minded persons had to pause for a moment before they could heartily approve of so strange and bold a proceeding as this appeared to be'.[4] It seemed at first sight as if 'the might of human science were coming into a positive and direct collision with Divine Power and Wisdom'. This was indeed matter for thought, in the days before Darwin. But Christianity, if such it was, gave ground very quickly. Simpson's arguments found an audience that was perhaps very ready to be persuaded, and the comfortable conclusion was soon reached that chloroform anaesthesia was 'only another instance of that most important truth, that human science is *not* opposed to the Divine decrees'.[5] What remained were powerful Victorian convictions about the nature and role of women and their proper place in a civilised society. The accepted view among educated people was that a woman should be good, loving, submissive, home-abiding, preferably beautiful, and married. The greatest poet of the age expressed it very clearly when he wrote

> God made the woman for the man
> And for the good and increase of the world.

Thus woman's true importance was that she submitted, and was a mother. Chloroform anaesthesia might or might not assist motherhood; but taking advantage of it did not, perhaps, look very like submission. What would women be up to next? Painless child-birth was not as harmless as it appeared; many saw it as a profound and disturbing change in essential social relationships, and probably felt that, in some obscure way, it heralded greater changes still (as perhaps it did). To this day medicine has gone on changing the place of women in society, and altering their lives far more than the lives of men.

It might be supposed that adapting to one new idea would have made the profession more ready to adapt to another; but there is no sign that Lister benefited from Simpson having preceded him. Three great difficulties prevented the ready adoption of antiseptic surgery. The first, as with chloroform anaesthesia, was the difficulty so many medical men found in carrying out the procedures correctly. There was more excuse for this in antisepsis than in chloroform anaesthesia. Lister's was an innovation not altogether easy to imitate. It was a complicated technique, not a standardised formula, and it was therefore essential to read Lister's descriptions of the method very carefully and in their entirety. There is ample evidence that this was often not done. Nor is this surprising, because those who object to a new plan or policy frequently fail even to understand it correctly; excitement dims perception. Moreoover, Lister kept changing the procedures. Some of the changes were easy to understand, but were nonetheless surprising. The *Lancet* was hardly to be blamed for its querulous observation in 1874, for example, that 'with every public appearance Professor Lister's carbolic solutions grow weaker and weaker while his faith grows more and more'. In addition, to deviate in only one particular from the recommended method might ruin everything. It remains true, however, that the profession showed remarkable incompetence in following Lister's instructions, and Lister's later attitude, that explanation was useless and that only those whom he instructed personally could be relied upon to become real antiseptic surgeons, is understandable. But the difficulty found by so many in doing what Lister recommended, and the consequent 'failures' that were held to prove the uselessness of antisepsis, were bound up with a second difficulty. This was, that antiseptic surgery depended on a theory. Those who did not understand or accept the theory and who nevertheless tried to follow antiseptic procedures were liable to constant mistakes, because they were not guided by the rationale of what they were doing. As Syme said at the start, the practice 'must be carefully studied and fully understood, theoretically as well as practically';[6] but the germ theory was too advanced for most of the British profession in the 1860s. The trouble here was, not that the new practice was based on insufficient science (as could have been said about anaesthesia) but that it was based on too much. This was the foundation of a shrewd contemporary observation:

> The truth is, that this is a question in science rather than in surgery, and hence, while eagerly adopted by the scientific Germans, and a little grudgingly by the semi-scientific Scotch, the antiseptic doctrine has never been in any degree appreciated or understood by the plodding and practical English surgeon. Happily for his patients, he has for a long time been to a considerable extent practicing a partially antiseptic system, thanks to his cleanly English instincts; but it has been like the lady who talked prose without knowing it.[7]

Whether or not English surgeons, not to mention hospital managers and nursing staff, had 'cleanly English instincts' and whether these were in any case cleanly enough to have been a good substitute for antisepsis might well be disputed; but the general argument of the first sentence is entirely sound. Lister was a hero in Germany long before he obtained much recognition in England, and in Scotland medical education, not least the scientific foundations of that education, was much superior to anything obtainable in England until at any rate 1870 or later.

The third ground of resistance to antiseptic surgery was perhaps the most important of all. This was, that it brought with it the likelihood, even the certainty, of extensive and in part unforeseeable changes in the practice of surgery, and could thus be viewed as a fundamental threat to the qualifications, attainments, earning capacity and social position of all who were expert in the 'old' surgery. What was at first seen as yet another new proposal for the dressing of wounds was in fact a proposal that was to change surgery almost out of recognition. The title of 'revolutionary innovation', so readily bestowed, is not so often deserved; but few innovations have been more truly revolutionary than Lister's. Before him, what was exclusively admired and valued was operative dexterity, and even as late as the 1870s (although chloroform had made this far less important) speed of work. For example, Sir Hector Cameron records an operation by Syme on a patient who had been stabbed in the neck in a public-house brawl; blood was escaping from the carotid artery and forming a swelling in the neck, and a fatal haemorrhage seemed imminent.

Syme decided to operate, to try to save two lives, the life of the patient and the life of his assailant who was in custody. The operating theatre was crowded. Lister's brow, while he stood waiting to assist, as always on such occasions, was bedewed with drops of sweat. The onlookers saw Syme make a long incision and cut boldly downwards. The blood spurted in jets and welled up everywhere. Syme's hands were buried in the depths of the wound, with a ligature held on a curved needle. Every now and then [the onlookers] glanced at the face of the patient, expecting at any moment to see the abrupt pallor of death spread over it. Suddenly Syme straightened himself; they could see that the haemorrhage had ceased, and a burst of applause and a buzz of excited conversation took place of the tense and awed silence.[8]

This was what a great surgeon was admired for; he was not unlike a batsman who scores a century in a test match, in the shortest possible time. He was in the centre of the action. What happened to the patient once the knives were put away was not considered to be much to the credit or discredit of the surgeon; the operation over, he washed his hands and went home. Lister changed this completely. What was now wanted was very careful, not spectacular, surgery, and as much attention to the patient after the operation as during it. Even as late as 1879 the idea that 'the discharges collecting in and around the wound are detrimental to the patient' sounded rather novel to the *Lancet;* but this was now to be central to surgery, not peripheral, and success now began to depend, as Lister himself put it, 'upon scrupulous attention to detail'. The change that took place can be personified. The 'ideal' surgeon before antisepsis was Liston: tall, powerfully built with strong hands, energetic, forthright, bold, a master of anatomy; but after the 1870s the Liston model had to be replaced as the surgeon's ideal by someone different — someone in fact much more like Lister himself: gentle, careful, patient, not necessarily a great manipulative surgeon, knowledgeable not only in anatomy but in pathology as well.

This change — or threatened change, as it at first was — must have been deeply repugnant to many established operators. Those who did not accept the germ theory, that is to say the great majority of surgeons, could not see the necessity for change, and felt that surgery was being made wearisome (the word was used several times to describe Lister's methods), that they were being asked to turn themselves into surgical nurses or even nursemaids, men of gauze and bandages, molly-coddlers of patients. It was not simply a matter of changing one's practice; acceptance of an almost new role was required. Those who prided themselves on their skill as operators felt demoted; 'an antiseptic spray', one of them defiantly remarked, 'would not compensaté for want of manipulative dexterity'. And there was another difficulty. Antiseptic surgery made possible a whole new range of operations; as Lister said in 1873, surgeons could now 'undertake with confidence operative procedures which, without efficient antiseptic measures, would be simply homicidal'. But this meant learning, and put the latest recruits to the profession on a par with their seniors. It tended to place, as Lawson Tait said, skilled and unskilled on a common level. And none of this was welcome to those whose position depended on the old techniques and the old skills. Of course there were established surgeons who were willing and able to adapt. But not everyone could be a James Syme, who at the age of 68 welcomed the antiseptic treatment on its first introduction, and observed with composure that 'it is certainly destined in no small degree to revolutionise the practice of surgery'.[9]

Besides these major reasons for trying to maintain the *status quo* there were other considerations which, although less important, had a significant influence. An obvious one was the personality of the participants. Simpson was an outstanding man in any company. Ambitious to excel, enormously energetic, very widely read, kindly (unless crossed), ingenious, gregarious, combative — even aggressive; a very human man, he had, it was said, no acquaintances, only friends. But he also had enemies. He was unscrupulous in controversy; possessed, and used, powers of abusive rhetoric that were outstanding even in an age of abusive rhetoric, and, not ashamed of his origin as 'a poor baker's son', never pretended to be a well-spoken, genteel, orthodox supporter of the medical establishment. Neither for that matter, did Lister; but Lister was peculiar in a quite different way. He inherited wealth, and could have become an eminent London surgeon with a lucrative practice. But he was by inclination a scientist in a profession that did not, when he was a young man, have much to do with science; surgeons least of all. He did research, which was strange, and went from London to Scotland, which was perhaps even stranger. And if Simpson had no acquaintances, only friends, Lister had no friends, only acquaintances. He inspired respect in everyone; but he could not receive affection. He was a solitary figure; and until almost the end of his campaign for antisepsis he spoke as such. These facts are important, because in a small world such as medicine was at that time, personalities matter. Findings are not simply findings; they are the findings of someone. The reputation of the author may affect their credibility; his personality and connections, in a small world, may affect their acceptability.

Simpson made many enemies, Lister no friends; and the consequences for the spread of their ideas were considerable. It may be said that this is merely a historical curiosity, that life is different today; the field of science and its population has become larger, and therefore more objective, less personal. But perhaps that would require to be proved. For example, would Watson and Crick have reacted in quite the same way if the erroneous solution to the DNA problem proposed in 1953 had been put forward by someone other than the great Linus Pauling?

Connected with personality was the force of national sentiment. Simpson was, by origin, education, manner, accent and everything else, a Scotsman; and he never worked outside Edinburgh. Lister was an Englishman, and a wealthy one at that; but he was also originally a Quaker, which set him a little apart, and he worked in Scotland for so long, from 1852-77 without a break, that in the eyes of his contemporaries he became completely identified with Scottish medicine. This mattered, because there was division and rivalry, not so much between England and Scotland, as between London and Scotland, especially between London and Edinburgh. Edinburgh was the most famous, perhaps one should say, the only famous medical school in Britain. Innumerable distinguished doctors and surgeons who achieved fame and fortune in England in the first half of the nineteenth century came from Scotland, most of them from Edinburgh. They outshone, if they did not actually outnumber, their English colleagues. The Royal Colleges in London, to put it mildly, disliked this domination by the Scots. For example, when Sir James Clark, born in Cullen and educated at Aberdeen and Edinburgh, was appointed as physician to Queen Victoria in 1837 the Fellows of the exclusive Royal College of Physicians 'looked on the appointment of a northern graduate very much as the bench of bishops might resent the intrusion of a Dissenter'.[10] This attitude delayed acceptance, certainly in London, of chloroform anaesthesia in midwifery. If Simpson had not lectured his colleagues so forcefully on the wickedness of not using chloroform, some of the London obstetricians might have been slower in finding arguments against it. And when Lister's turn came, the fact that Edinburgh had pioneered and triumphed in 1847-55 must have strengthened resistance to yet another new idea from north of the border.

In one other way, and much more clearly, the work of Simson interacted with that of Lister. Simpson is remembered for his one great contribution, chloroform anaesthesia; but he also initiated the hospitalism controversy. That controversy is almost forgotten, and Simpson's admirers tend to regard his part in it as best forgotten. In concentrating a battery of largely worthless statistics on the relation between surgical mortality and the size of hospitals Simpson seemed to miss the point. But in fact he made it inescapable. Without Simpson there would have been no controversy, and without the controversy the hospitals would have remained far more unhealthy places than they actually were by the last quarter of the nineteenth century. They would have been more overcrowded, worse ventilated, and dirtier, and the death rate in them would accordingly have been higher. So far so good. But the fact that better hospital hygiene was lowering the death rate at the same time that antisepsis was coming into use greatly confused the mind of the profession. If the death rate shown by 'non-Listerian' surgeons had remained constant while that shown by 'Listerian' surgeons fell, the case for antisepsis would have been obvious. But part of the trouble was, that both rates fell together. In time, it became clear that the 'Listerians' were doing better; and also, in time, it became clear that the germ theory of disease, which was the scientific basis of their procedures, had to be accepted. But ten years and more were required for the truth to be perceived. Good statistics and careful analysis of them would soon have separated out the two causes of the one effect, and would have helped to prove Lister's case; but these statistics were not available. As for the germ theory, it made slow headway in England. So most surgeons continued to work on an empirical basis, and were actually impeded by the fact that two valuable innovations, and not just one, came into use at about the same time. In a sense, Lister had to compete with better hospital hygiene, and to convince his antiseptic surgery an unnecessary and tiresome expense.

Can anything more general be said about the innovation process on the basis of these two, or hospitalism is included, three instances? The number is paltry, but the cases themselves are of exceptional importance, and they are very well documented. It may therefore not be too foolhardy to try to extract one or two points of possibly wider interest from the preceding assemblage of evidence and argument. But there are two caveats.

First, all medical innovation may be a special case. This is because medicine, while constantly changing, naturally resists change. There are often good reasons for this. Surgeons and physicians have always been reluctant to risk the well-being of their patients by trying something new, something that is recommended but not known; they hesitate, for the best of reasons, to take what is perhaps a newcomer's word for it, to experiment upon their patients. Also, medicine is not an exact science. Every case is unique and the data are poor. In these circumstances what counts enormously is experience. This experience is both cumulative — the tradition of successful customary practice — and personal in the senior members of the profession. The force of the past and the authority of the establishment are both unusually great in medicine. Both operate to safeguard the patient from untried ideas even when the more venturesome in the profession have overcome their scruples and are willing to experiment a little. Thus in 1872 Sir William Fergusson, whom Lister succeeded as Professor of Surgery at King's College Hospital and who was a very distinguished exponent of many of the new and important developments in conservative surgery, observed that there were 'strange views afloat' regarding the accepted Hunterian doctrines relating to inflammation,

> most notably in this respect, that what Hunter thought was developed by Nature from within, is now alleged to have origin in external influences and agencies . . . Gentlemen, there must ever be theories in surgery as in medicine, and when these are propounded by men of undoubted character and consideration, it behoves us all to wait cautiously to see the influence of time in the development of facts for or against what may be called the fashionable doctrines of the day.[11]

But medicine cannot propose to be immune from change; and caution can go too far. The past santified no new ideas, and older men often cannot change their ways of thinking even when there are 'facts' a-plenty.

Secondly, it is all too easy to sit in judgement on the past. Thus it is tempting to pose the question, was the adoption of chloroform anaesthesia into medical practice, in surgery and in midwifery, commendably rapid or deplorably slow? Questions of this kind are often asked and often answered; but what meaning they have, if any, is not always clear. There is the difficulty, first, of knowing exactly what is meant by 'adoption into practice'. How much adoption are we talking about? In the case of one innovation, for example, a minority of practitioners may adopt it almost at once, it then spreads slowly but steadily and is in general use in ten years; in another case, a new idea may have no immediate impact for several years but be in general use within say, five or six years of its introduction. It is not obvious which of these innovations is 'adopted' more rapidly than the other. Quite apart from this difficulty there remain further problems regarding the criteria by which speed of adoption is to be judged. In the case of chloroform anaesthesia not everyone was agreed that the reduction of pain was a major objective. Many doctors who took part in the controversy regarded pain as not particularly important, or even as salutary, and because such opinions sometimes reflected judgments of value about what is good and what is evil, it is impossible to describe the delay in adopting chloroform as blameworthy or not without first making a judgment on these moral judgments themselves. From a present-day point of view the general adoption of chloroform in midwifery was lamentably slow; but if one takes the position that no patient's life should be risked in any way except to avoid extreme and destructive pain, it is perfectly possible to argue that the process of adoption was inexcusably rapid. Of course, not all opposition to chloroform anaesthesia was of this kind. Some opposition was based on refusal to examine the evidence, based, that is to say, on believing what was even at that time demonstrably untrue. Delay through misunderstanding and ignorance can be called blameworthy, and in so far as this was what held up the adoption of chloroform anaesthesia the process can fairly be condemned as slow. But it is impossible to determine how much delay was of this kind. And therefore, for all these reasons, there is little to be gained in categorising the adoption of innovations in medicine as either fast or slow.

To ask in a general way what assists and what impedes innovation may nevertheless be instructive. On the face of it, and assuming that what is proposed will, in time, be recognised as a genuine improvement, what matters is:

(A) *the idea itself*; some ideas are more complicated than others, or seem less surprising, or relate more closely to the old technology, etc:

(B) *the capacity and willingness of the audience to adopt the idea*; innovation is a social process, and an audience may be more or **less** geared, by training and/or habit, to understand, appreciate **and** adopt new ideas.

But obviously what is summarised in this way is a very complicated matter. Previous chapters have shown that the reception given to Simpson's and Lister's path-breaking proposals was the outcome of many kinds of influence and consideration, and that, certainly in these two cases, B should be broken down into sub-sections as follows:

(B) 1. the capacity to understand and to imitate;

2. the likelihood that what is proposed, although it may be an improvement on the whole, carries with it some disadvantages which may not at first be apparent, which may require to be assessed, or which may make the innovation undesirable or inapplicable in certain situations;

3. the implications, not strictly or not at all scientific, which the idea has for those adopting it; that is to say, adoption may affect job prospects, or earning capacity, or the need to re-train, etc;

4. the implications of adoption for what is done or thought outside the area immediately concerned; these implications are likely to be moral, political or economic, and may thus spread very wide;

5. the personalities and position of those who might give a lead in adoption;

6. national or local sentiment.

And there is also, conversely, the ability of the innovator to put his ideas forward in a lucid and persuasive way. This aspect of the matter may also be broken down, as follows:

(C) 1. the capacity to explain and persuade;

2. the loneliness or otherwise of the innovator; that is to say, has he or has he not at an early stage the active support of colleagues, preferably of colleagues who themselves make some contribution, even if only a small one, to the idea?

3. the personality and position of the innovator.

This rough schema could be extended and refined, but it is adequate to bring out the fact that social considerations can much more easily be listed than scientific ones; of the ten points listed under A to C, only two are wholly or even largely a matter of science: A and B2. Admittedly, the distinction between science (what is known) and the scientist (the person who knows) cannot be absolute. Thus B1. and C1. could also reasonably be regarded as matters of science. But they are not wholly matters of science in a straightforward sense, and are to some extent, and the remaining six points are entirely, social considerations.

Taken by itself, this may not be very impressive. An analysis showing a preponderance of social as opposed to scientific considerations can always be secured by lumping all the scientific considerations together and listing the several social considerations separately from one another. Also, one matter of science may outweigh in importance all the social factors in sight. This was perhaps the case with chloroform anaesthesia and antiseptic surgery, because the ideas of both Simpson and Lister were open to serious scientific criticism and practical objection. Thus Simpson's opponents were perfectly correct in saying that the action of chloroform was mysterious, that it was therefore dangerous to use, and that needless risks were likely to be taken. What was proposed, they truly said, was something not thoroughly understood — although the response has to be that in those days there was very little in medicine that was thoroughly understood. In the case of Lister's work, the objections were, in a way, more serious. The earliest versions of antiseptic surgery were from a practical point of view, extremely crude. Moreover, because antiseptic surgery was founded on a theory, it was open to theoretical attack. Lister's ideas of microbiology, were, inevitably, rudimentary and in some respects erroneous. In particular, he had virtually no idea even in 1880 of the vast variety of bacteria in existence and hence greatly exaggerated the probability of morbific germs being present in significant numbers in a normal atmosphere; he was unaware, until after 1880, of the extent to which damaged tissue is the ideal medium for multiplying germs, having no blood supply to provide oxygen; he probably underestimated the importance of sterilising the skin in order to get rid of staphylococci; and he did not realise the wide variations among different bacteria in their resistance to heat and antiseptics. Hence his own methods sometimes failed, he was unable to offer a satisfactory explanation of surgical success without antisepsis, and could not meet some of the objections of Bastian and others that, for example, morbific germs introduced into the bloodstream often produced no harmful effects. Consequently, his opponents were right in saying that however good Lister's operative results might be, his theories did not explain all the relevant facts. Nevertheless, the germ theory, even as then understood, had far more explanatory power than any of its rivals, and this fact was, in the end, decisive. Doubtless there is nothing exceptional in all this. It is probably true that one of the commonest features of new ideas — certainly of practical new ideas — is their imperfection. Few spring from the brain or the drawing board of the inventor without grave defects. The steam-engine, the motor-car, the typewriter, the hypodermic syringe; each, when first introduced, was a crude device full of flaws and limitations.

And yet, although scientific argument played a substantial part in delaying the introduction of chloroform anaesthesia and antiseptic surgery, the social forces at work were also very important. Personalities played a big part; so, demonstrably, did 'moral' arguments (in the case of chloroform anaesthesia), so did the threat to established professional security and career prospects (in the case of antisepsis); so, above all, did the capacity of the profession to understand and imitate. It would not be easy to maintain that straightforward scientific arguments outweighed all or any of these social factors in importance.

No doubt the reception accorded to every scientific innovation is different, just as every innovation is itself different. What happens to an innovation that is made in the realms of theory may be very different from what happens to an innovation that is made in the realms of practice. What happens in medicine may be very different from what happens in astronomy. What happened in the 1850s and 1860s and 1870s may be very different from anything that happens or that could happen in the 1970s. Undoubtedly, the competence, or rather the incompetence, of the medical profession in the mid-nineteenth century seems very strange today. But it may not be absurd to suggest that some fundamental characteristics of the reaction to Simpson's and to Lister's proposals may always be present in the reception accorded to new ideas; that to some extent *the nature of the argument may recur*.

There are two reasons why this is likely to be so. First, every innovation enters an already occupied world; that is to say, it appears as a new method of doing or helping to do something that was almost certainly, more or less, done before. (Calculations were done before computers; news and entertainment were disseminated long before radio or television.) Therefore an innovation is a change which probably displaces something. Far from having a free run, like a solitary horse frisking about in a meadow, a new idea has to make its way through the resisting medium of established ways of thinking and doing. These ways depended on past experience and past education, and these — part of the lives of everyone in the field concerned — are what must be challenged and disturbed. Thus the impact of an innovation can never be a matter simply of science or technology, although these aspects must be extremely important. It is also, and may be more immediately, a matter of institutions and human nature.

Secondly, the impact of an innovation depends crucially on the relevant system of education. Is that system in touch with the frontiers of new knowledge? Does it teach its pupils to think, or does it only teach them the received truths of the day? Medical education in England in the mid-nineteenth century quite obviously was most defective in both respects. Young men were taught to memorise the accepted answers to accepted questions, and thinking for oneself never came into it. (A good deal of university education, not only in medicine, is still precisely of this character.) The result was that men faced with a new idea reacted in the only way that was possible; they stuck to what they knew. They declared, or they implied, that the established practice which it was proposed to amend or replace was itself so satisfactory and successful as not to stand in need of reform; and all attempts to prove that the 'old method' was more objectionable, or more fatal, encountered what Simpson called 'stern denial and anxious contradition'. No doubt matters were made worse by the fact that medical education of that day had very little to do with research, and was instead founded on the authority of the past, often the remote past. Out of touch with any modern ideas, the profession found it doubly difficult to absorb and adapt to what was new and revolutionary.

In so far as medicine was changing before 1850, or before 1870, and medical education with it, the younger members of the profession should have been at an advantage over the older members; they should have been at least a little more in touch with the direction of new developments, even if they had no better a grasp of the methods of thought than their elders; and it is conventional to suppose that men under 40 are more innovative and adaptable than those who are nearer three score and ten – did not Newton say that at the age of 23 he was 'in the prime of my invention'? The anaesthesia case, however, does not do much to support the contention that youth is for innovation and age is against it. Admittedly, Simpson was only 36 when he discovered chloroform anaesthesia (a fact obscured by the many portraits and photographs of Simpson as a grand old man in middle age) and Snow at that date was only 34, and admittedly Robert Lee, who was a bitter opponent, was 54 and Meigs in Philadelphia was 55. But G.T. Gream, who was almost as conservative in his views as Lee, was in his early 30s, and Syme, who from the start lent his very influential support to the use of chloroform, was 48; the most startling of all, J.C. Warren in Massachusetts, who gave Morton his great opportunity in 1846 and who then very effectively supported the use of ether in operations, (he was in a good position to do so for he was the outstanding American surgeon of his day), was 68 in 1846. Thus there were young and old men on both sides of the fence. The antisepsis case presents a similar picture. Lister published his first paper on antisepsis when he was 40. The only surgeon of importance who gave him full support before the battle was nearly won was Syme, who was 68 in 1867. Men of influence who were sympathetic, although they had doubts about the method, were Gamgee (39 in 1867), Thomas Keith (40) and Spencer Wells (49). The senior members of the profession, except for Syme, were, at best, no help to Lister. Sir William Fergusson (59), a bold and skilful operator and 'the greatest practical surgeon of our time', according to Sir James Paget, would only wait and see. Sir James Paget himself (53) could not make out what the antiseptic method was. Thomas Nunneley, a strong opponent, was 58 in 1867. On the other hand, Sir John Eric Erichsen, who approved of cleanliness in hospitals but was to the end sceptical about antisepsis, was 49; and one of the most vocal, persistent, and effective of Lister's opponents — outstandingly successful, moreover, in his own surgical work — was Lawson Tait, who was only 22 in 1867. To make matters worse, Tait was a graduate of Edinburgh University. These facts neither support nor detract from the argument that youth and new ideas go together. Probably medicine and medical education changed so little between 1800 and 1850 that it made almost no difference whether a man graduated at the beginning or at the end of that period. Where a man was trained mattered more than when he was trained.

In any event, professional education seems to have been the dominant institutional factor in the battles for chloroform anaesthesia and antiseptic surgery; and so it probably is in all similar cases. And therefore, because new ideas have always to compete with established practice, and because adaptability always depends principally on education, there are two reactions to be found in all cases of innovation, in greater or lesser degree, and which have been illustrated in the preceding pages.

First, the members of the profession, poorly educated both young and old and thus little able to cope with new ideas, refused to look at the facts. This was done not so much by denying the truth of what was true as by asserting the truth of what was not true. Chloroform, it was alleged, retarded delivery, it caused convulsions, it affected the system for months after being administered; antiseptic surgery failed as often as it succeeded, it retarded recovery, it was based on the quite erroneous notion that spontaneous generation never took place. Countless examples of these and similar groundless assertions have already been given in preceding chapters. Only one more need be set down here, as a final sample. In 1856, the *Lancet* reported that 'when water . . . has been boiled or distilled . . . observers of eminence have declared that they have seen the debris of vegetable matter, while undergoing decomposition, transformed into infusoria'.[12] It must have been disheartening for the innovators, to say the least, to have the truth constantly disregarded and untruth persistently repeated. This may be why Simpson, despairing of the force of argument, declared that success could come only by experience, i.e. by the gradual accumulation of cases until the sheer weight of them could no longer be ignored. Converts had to be made gradually, because they did not wish to know. They did not wish to examine the facts, nor even have them brought to their notice. There is nothing unusual in this. The opponents of Galileo, as has been said, did not oppose him by looking through his telescope, nor the opponents of Newton by looking through his calculations.

Secondly, abandoning logic, men took refuge in emotion. The tone of medical debate in the nineteenth century was often extremely acrimonious, and the new discoveries certainly made it worse. The Edinburgh medical school was in a state of perpetual uproar and its members frequently abused one another in terms that would almost certainly land their present-day successors in court. 'It is only too sadly notorious', said Lawson Tait in 1871, 'that medical life in the Scotch metropolis is mixed up with personal polemics to a degree that is elsewhere unknown in civilised society'. But rancorous argument and abuse were not confined to Edinburgh; no one was safe. When John Snow denied, before the Committee on the Public Health and Nuisances Removal Bills, that blood poisoning could be caused by inhaling air contaminated by putrid matter, the *Lancet* wrote as follows:

> Dr Snow claims to have discovered that the law of the propagation of cholera is the drinking of sewage-water. His theory, of course, displaces all other theories [which] attribute great efficacy in the spread of cholera to bad drainage and atmospheric impurities . . . The fact is, that the well whence Dr Snow draws all sanitary truth is the main sewer. His *specus*, or den, is a drain . . . he has fallen down through a gully-hole and has never since been able to get out again.[13]

All this, and more, because Snow declined to say that bad smells could be a direct cause of blood poisoning. In this case the writer had nothing to gain for himself by believing what he wanted to believe; his object was simply the improvement of public health through the removal of tanneries and the like from the middle of densely populated areas. Abusive personal attacks have of course the advantage of distracting attention from logical argument. But in any case, when evidence and logic lead to an unwelcome  conclusion, frustration and anger are apt to be the result. And to make matters worse, it seems that abusive opposition to innovation may often be founded to some extent on calculations of personal gain or loss, although perhaps dimly perceived. In this case, the real objections may be unstated ones. The opposition to antisepsis was probably partially of this kind; experienced operators felt alarmed, because new operations would become possible, new skills be required, new men come to the fore. Apprehensive for themselves, they became excited, inaccurate and insulting.

Generalisation is always hazardous. In the course of history there may have been innovations that were welcomed by everyone; but it would be unreasonable for an innovator to expect a universal welcome. He must therefore be prepared for trouble. And the best way to overcome trouble is not to lecture and browbeat the unpersuaded, as Simpson tended to do, nor to expect the disinterested and passionless triumph of reason, as Lister seemed to do, but to look on innovation as a part of the endless process of education. To innovate is to educate. Having educated himself, the innovator must educate others. At this stage, what counts is not so much the innovation or the innovator as the world in which he has to work. The better educated the population, the easier the innovator's task. And this must be so, because the best-educated populations (not necessarily the most-educated) are the easiest to educate further, the most adaptable, the least apt for a flight into unreason; the most likely to understand and to appreciate the words of Bishop Berkeley: 'Everything is what it is and not another thing; why, then, do you wish to be deceived?'

## Notes

1. James DeBack, *The Discourse of James DeBack, Physician in Ordinary to the Town of Rotterdam* (London, 1673), quoted in B.J. Stern, *Society and Medical Progress* (Princeton, 1941), p. 185.

2. These examples of resistance to new ideas in medicine are elaborated in Stern, *Society and Medical Progress*, Chapter IX.

3. It is true that Simpson lost a patient under chloroform in 1860; but is very doubtful that he was killed by the anaesthetic.

4. *British and Foreign Medico-Chirurgical Review,* vol. II, (1848), p. 519.

5. Ibid.

6. *British Medical Journal*, vol. I, (1868), p. 1.

7. *Lancet*, vol. I, (1878), p. 36.

8. H.C. Cameron, *Joseph Lister the Friend of Man* (London, 1949), pp. 42–3.

9. *British Medical Journal*, vol. I, (1868), p. 371.

10. *Lancet*, vol. II, (1870), p. 66.
11. *Lancet*, vol. II, (1872), p. 190.
12. *Lancet*, vol. I, (1856), p. 1.
13. *Lancet*, vol. I, (1855), p. 635.

# APPENDIX

The following passage is to be found in Simpson's lecture notes 'Natural and Morbid Parturition', now in the library of the Royal College of Physicians in Edinburgh. The notes are dated 1843-4. The passage appears in Charles Merriman, *A Synopsis of the various kinds of Difficult Patrituition,* first published in London in 1814, and was taken by him from a work by M. Sacombe of Paris, who, says Merriman, had had the opportunity, 'however undecorously embraced, of witnessing the progress of a natural labour, not by the finger, but the eye.' The comment in the middle of the passage, in brackets, is also by Merriman.

### Note in Merriman's Cases of Difficult Parturition

June 11th 1781, a counsellor of the Court of Excise at Montpellier invited me to dine with him at his country house at Laverune, a village about a league distant from Montpellier. We were scarcely arrived, when we were informed that the daughter of his gardener, 16 years of age, tall and well made, was attacked with the first pains of labour.

The midwife of the village was dangerously ill, my friend therefore recommended me to supply her place, and in consequence I was willingly accepted by the patient.

The Pains were pretty active, and were directed towards the Os-uteri. Eager to avail myself of an opportunity so favourable for examining the secrets of Nature, and of seizing her, as it were, in the midst of her operations, I had a camp-bed prepared for the young woman in a large and airy room, where I alone was present with her. I was sure that I should not be interrupted in my observations. The girl's mother was at Montpellier; her husband had left home, early in the morning, to proceed to sea; the master of the house had no wish to witness the process of child-bearing; in short, I was destined, in the attendance on my patient, to be 'tête à tête' with Nature herself.

The situation and position of my patient were such, as easily allowed me to be a spectator of everything that passed, while she was altogether ignorant of the breach thus furtively made upon her modesty: and that I might neither be surprised, nor interrupted by her, in my observations, I hung up a curtain between us, under the pretence of preserving her from the rays of the sun, and from the teazing of the flies.

I ought to have observed that I should not have placed the patient in the bed, but the labour pains were very forcing, the os-uteri was dilated at every throe and approached the centre of the pelvis, the pulse was become quick, the countenance was flushed, her anxiety was constantly increasing; in a word, everything announced that the termination of the labour was approaching. Unless all these symptons of a speedy delivery are present, the woman in labour ought to be prevailed upon to walk about, because moderate exercise tends to induce the natural contractions of the uterus.

In this state of affairs, I took my station, watching everything attentively, and determined to leave everything to nature as much as if my patient had been alone, in the midst of a forest. Thus, with, if I may so say, a pair of compasses in my eye, a watch in one hand, and a pencil in the other, I witnessed the truly ravishing spectacle of a natural labour.

From 10 o'clock in the morning, precisely, till 11, the girl had seven pains, which progressively increased in force, and succeeded each other as follows:

| | | | Interval | Duration |
|---|---|---|---|---|
| Between the | 1st and | 2nd | pain there was an interval of 15 minutes and the pain lasted | 21 seconds. |
| between the | 2nd and | 3rd | 14 | 27 |
| | 3rd | 4th | 10 | 27 |
| | 4th | 5th | 8 | 29 |
| | 5th | 6th | 7 | 32 |
| | 6th | 7th | 6 | 35 |

From 11 o'clock till 12 the patient had 12 pains, progressively increasing in force and succeeded each other as follows:

| | | | Interval | Duration |
|---|---|---|---|---|
| Between the | 7th and | 8th | 6 | 36 |
| | 8th | 9th | 6 | 40 |
| | 9th | 10th | 6 | 42 |
| | 10th | 11th | 5 | 45 |
| | 11th | 12th | 6 | 45 |
| | 12th | 13th | 5 | 47 |
| | 13th | 14th | 5 | 49 |
| | 14th | 15th | 5 | 55 |
| | 15th | 16th | 4 | 62 |
| | 16th | 17th | 4 | 70 |
| | 17th | 18th | 4 | 87 |

|       |       | Interval |  | Duration |
|-------|-------|----------|--|----------|
| 18th  | 19th  | 4        |  | 93       |

The results from the observations are — 1st, that the interval between the pains is an inverse ratio to their duration; 2nd, that the duration of each pain is in direct ratio to their force; that is to say, that in proportion as the interval of pains diminishes, and in proportion as their duration increases, the force of each pain is progressively augmented.

The clock struck 12, the membranes burst, and the Liquor-Amnii was discharged with such violence as bedewed me from head to foot: and now, for the first time, I perceived the vermilion disc of that globe, which was about to thrust a new being into life. (There follows some of the fine writing before alluded to, comparing this spectacle to the glorious view of the morning sun, just rising above the Horizon etc. etc.).

At the 20th throe, which occasioned to the patient, a most acute expression of pain, the head of the child passed through the inferior aperture of the pelvis. This, I could easily judge to be the case, from the quivering of the external parts of generation, from the violent contraction of the genital muscles, and from the tension and protrusion of the perineum.

At the 21st pain, the head of the child passed through the external soft parts, the chin being turned towards the os-coecygis of the mother. The child remained in this situation about 5 minutes, when the 22nd pain came on, and gave to the body of the infant a new direction, turning the right shoulder towards the sacrum of the mother, and the left towards the symphisis pubis thus allowing them to pass through the long diameter of the inferior aperture of the pelvis. The head of the child described a circle of 90 degrees, the nose being at once turned towards the internal and middle part of the mother's left thigh.

This movement of rotation was a ray of light, which gave me more information respecting the mechanism of natural labour, than all the lessons that I had received from my masters.

The 23rd and last pain expelled the body of the child, which was received upon a cloth prepared for that purpose.

The placenta was expelled in 5 minutes after the birth of the child, being directed by the pain towards that thigh to which the child's face had been turned before.

The woman, fatigued by her pains and by the heat of the weather, sank into a sweet sleep, and rested an hour and a half.

# INDEX